T0263853

Evaluation of Sleep Complaints

Editor

CLETE A. KUSHIDA

SLEEP MEDICINE CLINICS

www.sleep.theclinics.com

Consulting Editor
TEOFILO LEE-CHIONG Jr

December 2014 • Volume 9 • Number 4

ELSEVIER

1600 John F. Kennedy Boulevard • Suite 1800 • Philadelphia, Pennsylvania, 19103-2899

http://www.theclinics.com

SLEEP MEDICINE CLINICS Volume 9, Number 4
December 2014, ISSN 1556-407X, ISBN-13: 978-0-323-32345-1

Editor: Patrick Manley
Developmental Editor: Barbara Cohen-Kligerman

Sleep Medicine Clinics (ISSN 1556-407X) is published quarterly by Elsevier Inc., 360 Park Avenue South, New York, NY 10010-1710. Months of issue are March, June, September and December. Business and Editorial Offices: 1600 John F. Kennedy Blvd., Ste. 1800, Philadelphia, PA 19103-2899. Customer Service Office: 3251 Riverport Lane, Maryland Heights, MO 63043. Periodicals postage paid at New York, NY and additional mailing offices. Subscription prices are $195.00 per year (US individuals), $95.00 (US residents), $406.00 (US institutions), $230.00 (Canadian individuals), $235.00 (international individuals), $135.00 (Canadian and international residents) and $452.00 (Canadian and international institutions). Foreign air speed delivery is included in all *Clinics* subscription prices. All prices are subject to change without notice. **POSTMASTER:** Send change of address to *Sleep Medicine Clinics*, Elsevier Health Sciences Division, Subscription Customer Service, 3251 Riverport Lane, Maryland Heights, MO 63043. Customer Service: **Tel: 1-800-654-2452 (U.S. and Canada); 314-447-8871 (outside U.S. and Canada). Fax: 314-447-8029. E-mail: journalscustomerservice-usa@elsevier.com (for print support); journalsonline support-usa@elsevier.com (for online support).**

Reprints. For copies of 100 or more of articles in this publication, please contact the Commercial Reprints Department, Elsevier Inc., 360 Park Avenue South, New York, NY 10010-1710. Tel.: 212-633-3874; Fax: 212-633-3820; E-mail: reprints@elsevier.com.

PROGRAM OBJECTIVE

The goal of *Sleep Clinics of North America* is to keep practicing physicians up to date with current clinical practice by providing timely articles reviewing the state of the art in patient care.

TARGET AUDIENCE

All practicing physicians and other healthcare professionals.

LEARNING OBJECTIVES

Upon completion of this activity, participants will be able to:

1. Discuss confusional arousals, nightmares, dream-enactment, sleep terrors and sleepwalking.
2. Review apneas, hypoventilation, snoring and irregular respiration.
3. Discuss movements during sleep including restless legs.

ACCREDITATION

The Elsevier Office of Continuing Medical Education (EOCME) is accredited by the Accreditation Council for Continuing Medical Education (ACCME) to provide continuing medical education for physicians.

The EOCME designates this enduring material for a maximum of 15 *AMA PRA Category 1 Credit*(s)™. Physicians should claim only the credit commensurate with the extent of their participation in the activity.

All other health care professionals requesting continuing education credit for this enduring material will be issued a certificate of participation.

DISCLOSURE OF CONFLICTS OF INTEREST

The EOCME assesses conflict of interest with its instructors, faculty, planners, and other individuals who are in a position to control the content of CME activities. All relevant conflicts of interest that are identified are thoroughly vetted by EOCME for fair balance, scientific objectivity, and patient care recommendations. EOCME is committed to providing its learners with CME activities that promote improvements or quality in healthcare and not a specific proprietary business or a commercial interest.

The planning committee, staff, authors and editors listed below have identified no financial relationships or relationships to products or devices they or their spouse/life partner have with commercial interest related to the content of this CME activity:

Anne Batson, MSN, RN, FNP-BC, DNS student; Macario Camacho, MD; Éric Frenette, MD; Chad C. Hagen, MD; Kristen Helm; Brynne Hunter; Susan Imamura, MD; Vikas Jain, MD, FAASM, CCSH; Clete A. Kushida, MD, PhD; Emmanuelle Lapointe, MD; Sandy Lavery; Patrick Manley; Jill McNair; Mitchell G. Miglis, MD; Rahul R. Modi, MS, DNB; Mahalakshmi Narayanan; Olukayode O. Ogunrinde, MD; Brandon R. Peters, MD; Jason Valerio, MSc, MD, FRCPC; Robert E. Weir, MB BS, MRCOphth, MD; Mia Zaharna, MD, MPH.

The planning committee, staff, authors and editors listed below have identified financial relationships or relationships to products or devices they or their spouse/life partner have with commercial interest related to the content of this CME activity:

Scott Leibowitz, MD, DABSM, FAASM is on speakers bureau for Jazz Pharmaceuticals plc.

UNAPPROVED/OFF-LABEL USE DISCLOSURE

The EOCME requires CME faculty to disclose to the participants:

1. When products or procedures being discussed are off-label, unlabelled, experimental, and/or investigational (not US Food and Drug Administration [FDA] approved); and
2. Any limitations on the information presented, such as data that are preliminary or that represent ongoing research, interim analyses, and/or unsupported opinions. Faculty may discuss information about pharmaceutical agents that is outside of FDA-approved labelling. This information is intended solely for CME and is not intended to promote off-label use of these medications. If you have any questions, contact the medical affairs department of the manufacturer for the most recent prescribing information.

TO ENROLL

To enroll in the Sleep Medicines Clinic Continuing Medical Education program, call customer service at 1-800-654-2452 or sign up online at http://www.theclinics.com/home/cme. The CME program is available to subscribers for an additional annual fee of USD $140.

METHOD OF PARTICIPATION

In order to claim credit, participants must complete the following:

1. Complete enrolment as indicated above.
2. Read the activity.
3. Complete the CME Test and Evaluation. Participants must achieve a score of 70% on the test. All CME Tests and Evaluations must be completed online.

CME INQUIRIES/SPECIAL NEEDS

For all CME inquiries or special needs, please contact elsevierCME@elsevier.com.

SLEEP MEDICINE CLINICS

FORTHCOMING ISSUES

March 2015
Sleep and Psychiatry in Adults
John Herman and Max Hirshkowitz, *Editors*

June 2015
Sleep and Psychiatry in Children
John Herman and Max Hirshkowitz, *Editors*

September 2015
Restless Legs Syndrome and Movement Disorders
Denise Sharon, *Editor*

RECENT ISSUES

September 2014
Sleep Hypoventilation: A State-of-the-Art Overview
Babak Mokhlesi, *Editor*

June 2014
Behavioral Aspects of Sleep Problems in Childhood and Adolescence
Judith A. Owens, *Editor*

March 2014
Central Sleep Apnea
Peter C. Gay, *Editor*

ISSUES OF RELATED INTEREST

Clinics in Chest Medicine, Vol. 35, No. 3 (September 2014)
Sleep-Disordered Breathing: Beyond Obstructive Sleep Apnea
Carolyn M. D'Ambrosio, *Editor*

Contributors

CONSULTING EDITOR

TEOFILO LEE-CHIONG Jr, MD
Professor of Medicine, Division of Pulmonary, Critical Care and Sleep Medicine, Department of Medicine, National Jewish Health, University of Colorado, Denver, Colorado; Chief Medical Liaison, Philips Respironics, Pennsylvania

EDITOR

CLETE A. KUSHIDA, MD, PhD
Director, Stanford University Center for Human Sleep Research; Professor, Department of Psychiatry and Behavioral Sciences; President, World Sleep Federation; Neurologist and Medical Director, Stanford Sleep Medicine Center, Stanford University Medical Center, Redwood City, California

AUTHORS

ANNE BATSON, MSN, RN, FNP-BC
DNS Student, The Sleep Medicine Practice, Laureate Medical Group, Northside Hospital, Atlanta, Georgia; Wellstar School of Nursing, Kennesaw State University, Kennesaw, Georgia

MACARIO CAMACHO, MD
Sleep Surgery and Medicine Division, Department of Otolaryngology-Head and Neck Surgery, Tripler Army Medical Center, Honolulu, Hawaii

ÉRIC FRENETTE, MD
Neurologist and Sleep Specialist, Department of Neurology, Centre Hospitalier Universitaire de Sherbrooke (CHUS), Assistant Professor of Neurology, Université de Sherbrooke, Sherbrooke, Québec, Canada

CHAD C. HAGEN, MD
Assistant Professor, Department of Psychiatry; Director, Sleep Disorders Program, Oregon Health and Science University, Portland, Oregon

SUSAN IMAMURA, MD
Department of Sleep Medicine, The Permanente Medical Group, San Jose, California

VIKAS JAIN, MD, FAASM, CCSH
Sleep Medicine, Oklahoma City, Oklahoma; Adjunct Clinical Instructor, Stanford University, Stanford

CLETE A. KUSHIDA, MD, PhD
Director, Stanford University Center for Human Sleep Research; Professor, Department of Psychiatry and Behavioral Sciences; President, World Sleep Federation; Neurologist and Medical Director, Stanford Sleep Medicine Center, Stanford University Medical Center, Redwood City, California

EMMANUELLE LAPOINTE, MD
Neurology Resident, Department of Neurology, Centre Hospitalier Universitaire de Sherbrooke (CHUS), Sherbrooke, Québec, Canada

SCOTT LEIBOWITZ, MD, D,ABSM, FAASM
The Sleep Medicine Practice, Laureate Medical Group, Northside Hospital; Department of Psychiatry and Behavioral Sciences, Emory University, Atlanta, Georgia

MITCHELL G. MIGLIS, MD
Clinical Instructor, Sleep Medicine, Neurology, Stanford University, Palo Alto, California; Department of Neurology, Stanford Sleep Medicine Center, Redwood City, California

RAHUL R. MODI, MS, DNB
Assistant Professor, Department of Otolaryngology-Head & Neck Surgery, Bharati Vidyapeeth Deemed University Medical College, Pune, India; Visiting Assistant Professor, Division of Sleep Surgery, Department of Otolaryngology-Head & Neck Surgery, Stanford University Medical Center, Redwood City, California

OLUKAYODE O. OGUNRINDE, MD
Sleep Specialist, Department of Sleep Medicine, Northwest Permanente, PC, Physician and Surgeons, Kaiser Permanente Health System, Salem, Oregon

BRANDON R. PETERS, MD
Consulting Assistant Professor, Department of Psychiatry and Behavioral Sciences, Stanford University, Novato, California

JASON VALERIO, MSc, MD, FRCPC
Division of Neurology, Department of Medicine, UBC Health Sciences Center Hospital, Vancouver, British Columbia, Canada

ROBERT E. WEIR, MB BS, MRCOphth, MD
Sleep Medicine Fellow, Sleep Disorders Program, Portland VA Medical Center, Oregon Health and Science University, Portland, Oregon

MIA ZAHARNA, MD, MPH
Sleep Medicine Physician, Kaiser San Jose Division of Sleep Medicine, The Permanente Medical Group, Inc, San Jose, California

Contents

Preface
Evaluation of Sleep Complaints

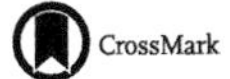

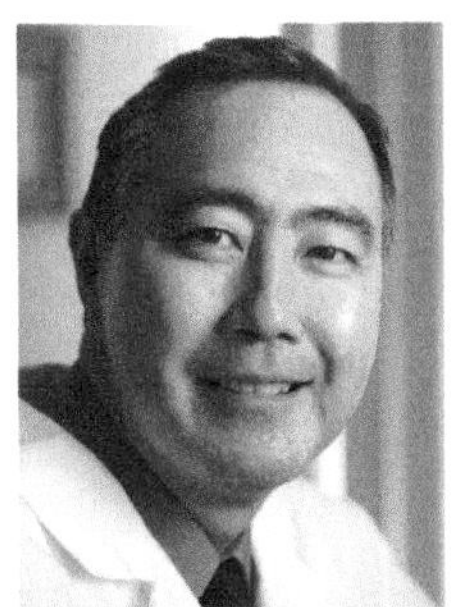

Clete A. Kushida, MD, PhD
Editor

This issue on the evaluation of sleep complaints would not have been possible without the outstanding contributions of a talented group of authors; their detailed and comprehensive articles will undoubtedly benefit any student, trainee, or clinician.

This work is divided into common sleep complaints, such as difficulty falling or staying asleep, which are symptomatic of the insomnias; irregular bedtimes and awakenings, jet lag, and shift work that may be associated with a circadian rhythm sleep disorder; daytime sleepiness, which can represent insufficient sleep but may also be associated with sleep, medical, and/or psychiatric disorders; snoring, irregular respiration, hypoventilation, and apneas, which are the main symptoms and signs of sleep-related breathing disorders; restless legs and periodic or rhythmic movements during sleep that characterize sleep-related movement disorders; confusional arousals, sleep terrors, sleepwalking, nightmares, and dream-enactment behaviors that are associated with parasomnias or unusual movement or behaviors during sleep; and poor sleep with age.

I am deeply indebted to the renowned and true pioneers of the field of sleep, William Dement, Christian Guilleminault, Sonia Ancoli-Israel, Chris Gillin, and Allan Rechtschaffen, who served as my mentors through various stages of my career. In all of my endeavors, I can always count on my parents, Samiko and the late Hiroshi Kushida, to assist me; this issue was no exception. This issue is dedicated not only to my parents and my wife, Shirley, but also to the marvelous teams of the NHLBI-sponsored Apnea Positive Pressure Long-Term Efficacy Study (APPLES), AHRQ-sponsored Comparative Outcomes Management with Electronic Data Technology (COMET), and PCORI-sponsored Sustainable Methods, Algorithms, and Research Tools for Delivering Optimal Care Study (SMART DOCS). I have been very fortunate to serve as principal investigator of these studies; key individuals from these studies include James Walsh, Pamela Hyde, Deborah Nichols, Kara Griffin, Eileen Leary, Rik Jadrnicek, Ric Miller, Tyson Holmes, Dan Bloch, Emmanuel Mignot, Rachel Manber, Chia-Yu Cardell, Rhonda Wong, Pete Silva, and Elyse Cohen, as well as NHLBI (Michael Twery and Gail Weinmann), AHRQ (Gurvaneet Randhawa), PCORI (Diane Bild), site directors, coordinators, consultants, committee members, data and safety monitoring board (DSMB) members, and other personnel without whom these projects could not have functioned in such a meticulous and efficient manner.

It is my sincere desire that the reader will strive to become an expert in the field of sleep medicine, and the first step toward this goal is

Sleep Med Clin 9 (2014) xi–xii
http://dx.doi.org/10.1016/j.jsmc.2014.08.010
1556-407X/14/$ – see front matter

the recognition of key sleep complaints, which will ultimately lead to the correct diagnosis and management of the underlying disorder. It is for this reason this issue was conceived, and, on behalf of the authors of this issue, we hope to have provided a resource that will stimulate further learning about the fascinating field of sleep medicine.

Clete A. Kushida, MD, PhD
Stanford Sleep Medicine Center
450 Broadway Street, 2nd Floor
Pavilion C MC 5704
Redwood City, CA 94063, USA

E-mail address:
clete@stanford.edu

Difficulty Falling or Staying Asleep

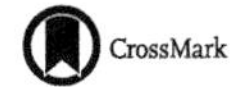

Scott Leibowitz, MD, D,ABSM[a,b,*], Anne Batson, MSN, RN, FNP-BC[a,c]

KEYWORDS

• Sleep maintenance • Excessive daytime somnolence • Sleep history • Insomnia
• Circadian rhythm disorders • Sleep-related breathing disorders • Actigraphy • Sleep testing

KEY POINTS

- Sleep complaints should be viewed as a symptom, not the problem, and a differential diagnosis list should be compiled based on the subtle features of these complaints.
- Screening tools and assessments are helpful in identifying and characterizing sleep complaints before or during the clinical encounter.
- An organized, systematic approach is preferred when evaluating patients' sleep complaints.
- Gathering specific core data points of the sleep history is crucial to accurately appreciate the nuances of patients' complaints and help to focus the differential diagnosis list.
- A firm understanding of the potential causes or exacerbating factors of the complaint is necessary to accurately guide the evaluation process.
- Several tools are available to help further characterize or diagnose conditions that may be responsible for patients' complaints.

INTRODUCTION

Sleep disorders are extremely common in the general population, and even more so when considering specific subpopulations. An estimated 50 million to 70 million US adults have sleep disorders.[1] Studies have shown that between 20% and 35% of adults report having 1 or more symptoms of insomnia and 10% to 20% have clinically significant insomnia syndrome.[2–6] Further, as many as 40% of patients more than the age of 60 years may experience insomnia, frequent nighttime awakenings, and disrupted sleep.[7] Extrapolated data from the Wisconsin Sleep Cohort Study estimated that the overall prevalence of obstructive sleep apnea was 9% for women and 24% for men.[8]

There are far-reaching consequences of untreated sleep disorders. Quality-of-life studies have shown the impact of sleep disorders on productivity, cognitive function, and work absenteeism.[9,10] Insomnia specifically has been shown to contribute to worsening psychiatric and health outcomes,[11,12] as well as having profound economic costs, with estimated total direct and indirect costs of $30 billion to $35 billion annually.[13] A recent investigation into the financial burden of the effects of insomnia provided estimates using data from 7428 US workers. Researchers reported that the annual loss in work performance is 367 million days, translating into a loss of US$ 91.7 billion.[14] Untreated obstructive sleep apnea has been linked to poor cardiovascular and metabolic disease outcomes.[15] A study in 2000 suggested that more than 800,000 drivers were involved in a motor vehicle accident as a consequence of sleep apnea. Those events cost 1400 lives and $15.8 billion.[16]

Disclosure: Dr S. Leibowitz is currently on the speaker's bureau for Jazz pharmaceuticals and has received honoraria. Mrs A. Batson has no conflicts to disclose.

[a] The Sleep Medicine Practice, Laureate Medical Group, Northside Hospital, 6135 Barfield Road NE, Atlanta, GA 30328, USA; [b] Department of Psychiatry and Behavioral Sciences, Emory University, 2004 Ridgewood Drive, Atlanta, GA 30322, USA; [c] Wellstar School of Nursing, Kennesaw State University, 1000 Chastain Road, Kennesaw, GA 30144, USA

* Corresponding author. 826 Hillpine Drive, Atlanta, GA 30306.
E-mail address: sleibowitz@laureatemed.com

Sleep Med Clin 9 (2014) 463–479
http://dx.doi.org/10.1016/j.jsmc.2014.08.005
1556-407X/14/$ – see front matter

The realization of the consequences to health coupled with the prevalence of these problems in Western society suggests that there should be a formal, structured sleep medicine curriculum embedded into the fabric of medical education. This curriculum would in turn produce physicians who are adequately prepared in the evaluation and treatment of sleep disorders on completion of their training. However, this has not been found to be the case.

According to a 2002 survey of more than 500 primary care physicians (PCPs) who self-reported their knowledge of sleep disorders, none reported their knowledge as excellent, 10% reported as having a good knowledge base, 60% reported a fair knowledge base, and 30% reported their knowledge as poor.[17] A survey in 1990 to 1991 of 37 American medical schools reported that sleep and sleep disorders were covered, on average, in less than 2 hours of total teaching time.[18] However, there is little to suggest that this trend has changed to any large extent. A 2007 review of medical specialty textbooks found that sleep and sleep disorders information made up approximately 2% of the content[19] and a study from 2011 found that only 3 hours of time were spent on sleep education as part of the core medical school curriculum.[20]

Insufficient training and knowledge of sleep disorders is likely a major contribution to underrecognition and undertreatment. A 2003 US poll found that 67% of adults more than 55 years of age reported having symptoms of sleep disorders at least a few nights a week, but only 13% had been formally diagnosed with a sleep condition, and only 9% had received treatment.[21] In the 2005 National Sleep Foundation's Sleep in America Poll, 70% of respondents reported that their doctors had never asked about their sleep habits.[22]

More structured, integrated education with regard to identification, evaluation, and management of sleep disorders during the process of medical training is therefore likely to increase awareness and vigilance about the identification of these conditions.

Patients with sleep disturbances should be approached using the same methodology taught to medical students to assess any chief complaint; that is, to identify the underlying condition responsible for the complaint, as opposed to reacting to and treating a symptom. If a sleep-related symptom is viewed as the problem, treatments directed toward the complaint will often be incomplete and fraught with complications and side effects. Although the complaints of difficulty falling asleep, waking frequently during the night, and difficulty reinitiating sleep are defining symptoms of insomnia, it is crucial to appreciate the multiple conditions that often share these as presenting symptoms. Symptom-directed treatment not only carries the risk of masking important and harmful conditions, but also often proves to be ineffective until such time that the underlying problem is addressed. As with any other complaint or problem, a thorough history and physical, followed by the generation of a complete differential diagnosis list, promotes a focused evaluation, and guides the treatment process in a safer, more precise, and more effective manner.

The common use of hypnotic sleep aids has gained recent attention after studies reported decreased levels of alertness while driving, prompting the US Food and Drug Administration to recommended lower doses of zolpidem for women.[23] The risks of prescription sleep aids have been well established.[24–27] A 2012 study that showed correlations between the ever use of benzodiazepines and a 50% increase in the risk of dementia mandates the judicious use of these medications.[28] Whether this relationship is causal does not negate the potential risk, and practitioners who are unable or unwilling to assess sleep complaints appropriately should think carefully before prescribing them.

However, to date, there has been little validation of a standardized, formally structured interview in a clinical setting for the evaluation of sleep complaints. Those studies that have been performed have not been reliably reproduced in large-scale, clinical settings.[29,30] Further, apart from sleep specialists, it is rare that clinicians have the time, resources, or training that are required to perform a comprehensive sleep evaluation for patients with these types of complaints. Nonetheless, having a better understanding and appreciation of the evaluation of sleep/wake complaints affords treating clinicians a broader knowledge of the appropriate management.

This article discusses these issues, describing in greater detail the barriers to care, approaches in identifying these patients, as well as an approach in the evaluation of patients complaining of difficulties initiating and maintaining sleep.

BARRIERS/ACCESS TO CARE

Insomnia is the most commonly reported sleep problem in the industrialized world but most insomniacs do not seek medical treatment. A 2005 study identified 3 main determinants to seeking care for sleep-related complaints: daytime fatigue (48%), psychological distress (40%), and physical discomfort (22%).[31] The high incidence of insomnia complaints paired with suboptimal recognition of the problem and tolerance by the patients leads to a gross underestimation of the negative outcomes of sleep disturbances.[32]

In the past, symptoms of sleep related breathing disorders (SRBD), which included snoring and excessive daytime somnolence, were not seen as indicators of a medical condition but rather as comical or annoying characteristics. Patients with sleep apnea were stereotyped as overweight, middle-aged, snoring men. Because of this perception, sleep apnea conditions were diagnosed incidentally during the perioperative period or during an evaluation of another medical condition such as a myocardial infarction. Diagnosis bias resulted because of the stereotype and created a barrier for referral for women, normal-weight adults, and the elderly.[28] A prospective cohort study in 2007 showed that, during primary care visits, only 19% of patients who scored high on the Berlin questionnaire, a screening tool shown to have a high predictive value for identifying individuals at high risk for sleep apnea, were referred for a sleep study.[33] To date, screening for obstructive sleep apnea is not a standard practice in the general physical examination.

ACCESS TO SLEEP SPECIALISTS

Board-certified sleep specialists (BCSSs) are not required to effectively evaluate sleep-related complaints; however, as in all specialties, there are advantages in having a BCSS perform the evaluation of patients with these complaints. BCSSs have a greater depth of understanding of the pathophysiology of sleep and wake disorders, diagnostic and treatment modalities, as well as the impact of comorbid medical conditions and medications on sleep/wake symptoms. Through this fund of knowledge, BCSSs are thus better able to generate a broader differential in terms of potential causes of sleep/wake symptoms. Studies have shown improved treatment outcomes in patients evaluated and managed by BCSSs specialists for obstructive sleep apnea.[34,35] Studies have also shown that specialized training in behavioral sleep medicine confers improved outcomes in patients with chronic insomnia.[36] A recent study from Australia showed that management of obstructive sleep apnea by PCPs was not inferior to management by specialists; however, extensive training and intensive nurse support was included in this trial. Such services are rarely, if ever, seen in clinical settings in primary care practices.[37]

However, access to BCSSs may be limited in certain areas of the country because of the limited numbers of specialists to date. Add to that the estimated 32 million Americans expected to enter the medical system with implementation of the Affordable Care Act (ACA), and access becomes an even greater issue.

Until the 1990s, board certification was unnecessary in order to practice sleep medicine. Only recently has qualification for board certification been achieved through the completion of a fellowship program accredited by the Accreditation Council for Graduate Medical Education. As a result, there exists a great deal of heterogeneity among specialists in terms of training as well as standards of practice. Further, as a by-product of the varied backgrounds of those clinicians with board certification in sleep medicine (eg, pulmonary medicine, internal medicine, neurology, otolaryngology), there exists the potential for biases and a limited frame of reference when evaluating patients with sleep and wake complaints. There is anecdotal evidence that there are several BCSSs who might be considered sleep apnea specialists as opposed to sleep specialists and with whom the evaluation of patients with sleep and wake complaints is distilled down to whether or not the patient has obstructive sleep apnea, rather than the focus being on determining the causes of their complaints. This widespread practice has clouded the perception of what the specialty encompasses, making referral to specialists in some areas less attractive.

Nonetheless, in the coming years, a collaboration between PCPs and BCSSs will be essential, the former being the first point of contact providing initial evaluation and management, with escalation to the BCSS for further management or in the event of uncertainty or a complicated initial presentation. Only with a firm knowledge of the many sleep disorders and representative complaints will this model be effectively used.

INITIAL ASSESSMENT

Initial evaluation of a sleep complaint can be misleading because the complaint has the potential to be both the symptom and the problem. In order to help differentiate this point, as well as to facilitate a more expedited encounter, the use of self-reported questionnaires and screening tools directed at identifying or characterizing potential causes of the complaints are helpful. These tools are preferably completed before the encounter so as to allow review by the treating clinician before or at the initial visit. There are numerous validated tools from which to use; however, it is important to choose instruments that characterize specific spheres of sleep and wake symptoms. Severity and duration of the complaint, weekday and weekend sleep habits, perceived daytime sleepiness, associated fatigue, mood disturbance, and cognitive dysfunction. Further, if the history is viewed as a sleep review of systems, patients are often able to characterize fairly accurately the nature of their symptom(s), allowing rapid differentiation between a symptom and a problem. However, there is no single tool or combinations of tools that have been systematically determined to be the most comprehensive and useful; however, there are several basic instruments that, when used together, help begin the process of formulating a differential diagnosis. **Table 1** lists for tools that are commonly used in the clinical setting.

Self-styled questionnaires are a simply means with which to screen for and rule out the presence of a variety of comorbid sleep disorders, medications, medical conditions, and psychiatric conditions that may be contributing to the symptom complex. It is crucial for the evaluating clinician to remember that symptoms such as excessive daytime somnolence, nighttime awakenings, and difficulties with initial sleep onset are not diagnostic of a problem, but are often a symptom as a result of a primary sleep disorder.

For example, studies have shown that more than 50% of patients with obstructive sleep apnea present with a complaint of insomnia.[38] Patients with circadian rhythm disorders by definition have difficulties with initial sleep onset or early morning awakenings, as well as daytime somnolence. Patients with restless legs syndrome and/or periodic limb movement disorder typically report sleep disturbances and often associated daytime consequences, as do patients with sleep-related breathing disorders. Individuals with chronic conditions that interfere with sleep, such as chronic pain, congestive heart failure, and lung disease, may set in motion a cycle of sleep disturbance. In these patients, it is important to determine whether the sleep-disrupting condition continues to be the driving factor behind the problem, or, as is the more common scenario, the sleep disturbance has become a primary disorder.[39]

With the multitude of sleep disorders and contributing influences that affect sleep and wake symptoms, the need for an organized, systematic approach to the evaluation of sleep-related complaints can be appreciated. As previously mentioned, there is not a validated, structured interview that can be referenced to direct this process; however, using a framework based on the knowledge of sleep and wake disorders and the subtle manifestations of each, an unstructured evaluation can yield a wealth of information to fully characterize the nature of an individual's problem, and, in so doing, inform the evaluation and management process. Using this conceptual framework to guide the initial evaluation, an integrated algorithm can be applied (**Fig. 1**).

THE INTERVIEW

The evaluation of sleep-related complaints should follow the same format as that taught for the evaluation of any medical complaint. This structure begins with identification of the chief complaint and then pursuit of the nuances of this complaint in terms of onset, duration, severity, and exacerbating and alleviating factors. This detailed characterization helps to contextualize the nature of the complaint and sift the differential diagnosis list down to a narrowed focus.

It is important to consider that the patient's chief complaint often contrasts starkly with the symptoms and problem. For example:

A 42-year-old man without a significant medical history presents to your office with the chief complaint of being unable to sleep. On accumulating the specifics of his history, he reports weekday and weekend bedtimes of 11 PM, and average wake times during the week of 6 AM with an alarm, and spontaneous weekend wake times of 8:30 AM. He describes initial sleep onset as rapid, but complains that he wakes frequently during the night, but generally without prolonged wake after sleep onset. He complains of nonrestorative sleep, daytime somnolence, unintentional napping most days on return home from work at 5 PM for 30 minutes, and intentionally on weekends in the midafternoon for 1 to 2 hours.

As is evident from this vignette, although this patient wakes frequently during the night, he has no difficulties with initial onset and rapid return to sleep after middle of the night awakenings. Although his chief complaint is that he cannot sleep, his primary symptom is of excessive daytime somnolence, with associated nighttime awakenings and nonrestorative sleep.

The process of exploring the subtleties of the symptoms in greater depth ultimately helps direct additional questioning and, if indicated, diagnostic testing. A patient who presents with isolated difficulties with initial sleep onset tends to have a narrower differential list than do middle of the night awakenings, early morning awakenings, and/or a combination of all 3 complaints.

Irrespective of the nature of the patient's complaint, gathering information regarding sleep/wake patterns and behaviors is essential in order to better characterize the nature of the complaints. This approach serves first to broaden and then focus the differential diagnosis list.

These data points should include weekend versus weekday bedtimes as well as lights-out time in both scenarios. Bedtime is often different than lights-out time, which may help to identify exacerbating maladaptive sleep behaviors. Time to fall asleep after lights out (sleep latency) is another important piece of information, as is frequency of nighttime awakenings, wake after sleep onset time/time to reinitiate sleep after awakenings, and intended final wake time. It is also important to differentiate final wake time from the vertical wake time; the latter implying that the patient is out of bed starting the day. Patients should attempt to estimate their average nightly total sleep times, perceived sleep quality, restfulness of sleep, and degree of daytime sleepiness. Characterizing frequency, duration, and timing of daytime naps and episodes of extreme sleepiness (which may not result in a nap) or unintended dozing helps to elucidate degree of sleepiness. Patients often underestimate their degree of sleepiness but may nap on a regular basis, suggesting a greater burden of sleepiness than was appreciated. Beyond these core points, screening for signs or symptoms that suggest a comorbid sleep disorder is crucial for the aforementioned reasons. Benefits, failures, or intolerance to previous treatments and previous diagnostic evaluation should be documented as well (**Box 1**).

DIFFICULTIES WITH INITIAL SLEEP ONSET

When evaluating a patient with sleep difficulties, attempts should be made to characterize approximate date of onset and to associate a possible precipitating event. If a clear association between a life event and the onset of symptoms exists, this often proves to be a combination of behavioral and biological factors mediating the problem (ie, psychophysiologic or primary insomnia). Individuals who have insomnia, be it early (initial sleep onset difficulties), middle (nighttime awakenings with prolonged wake after sleep onset), or late (early morning awakenings) have generally shown a vulnerability or a predisposition to these problems before the onset of the persistent problem in the form of transient episodes of insomnia.[40] Attempts should be made to elicit this prior history.

MODELS AND CAUSES OF INSOMNIA

Spielman and colleagues[41] proposed the 3-Ps model of insomnia, suggesting that individuals who have insomnia have predisposing traits for the development of insomnia, followed by a precipitating event that causes acute stress, pushing the individual over the so-called insomnia threshold. In response to the acute sleep difficulties, these individuals tend to engage in perpetuating behaviors that reinforce and condition these behaviors, creating the chronic problem.[42] These perpetuating factors tend to be maladaptive, sleep-prohibitive behaviors that generally impede initiation of sleep, and, over time, become the conditioned presleep behavior. These behaviors generally begin with poor sleep hygiene, which is often a compensatory response on the patient's part to cope with the sleep difficulties. These behaviors include variable bedtimes and wake times, prolonged time spent in bed awake (often in a failed attempt to increase the opportunity to sleep), engaging in waking behaviors (eg, watching television, reading, working on computers and mobile devices), as well as excessive caffeine intake, and napping.[43] Failed attempts at initiating sleep generally lead to maladaptive sleep thoughts in the form of catastrophizing the consequences of sleep loss, which elicits an anxiety response, which engages the central nervous system (CNS) waking mechanism and further impedes sleep onset. These so-called perpetuating factors have been proposed to be the driving force transitioning transient insomnia to a chronic problem.[41]

Identifying these behaviors is an important first step in diagnosing the condition responsible for the presenting symptoms and they also must be rectified as a component of the treatment process (**Box 2**). However, correcting sleep hygiene problems alone has not proved to be an effective stand-alone treatment of insomnia; rather, these issues must be resolved in conjunction with other treatment modalities in order to effectively resolve this problem.[39]

Characterizing medical problems that interfere with sleep onset, particularly chronic pain conditions or restless legs syndrome, is an obvious but often overlooked aspect of the history. Medications also have the potential to affect sleep onset. The presence and timing of activating medications such as selective serotonin reuptake inhibitors, stimulants, decongestants, and β-blockers should be discovered.

AROUSAL SYSTEM OVERACTIVITY

Studies have suggested that patients with insomnia have failure of their arousal systems to decline in activity with transition from waking to sleeping states, and generally are in a hyperaroused state both during wake and sleep.[44] This hyperarousal tends to manifest phenotypically in patients with chronic insomnia as a failure to experience sleepiness, but most patients with chronic insomnia tend to complain primarily of fatigue.[45] Differentiating these two symptoms is important because it may help to identify the

Table 1
Tools commonly used in the clinical setting

Self-reported Questionnaire	Description	Comments
Cleveland Sleep Habits Questionnaire	A 2-page instrument consisting of the Berlin and STOP portion of the STOP BANG to screen for OSA as well as the Epworth to screen for sleepiness Includes scoring instructions for ease of use	Additional single items have been added to screen for RLS, alcohol use, and narcolepsy Has been studied in primary care setting as a 1-use screening instrument[75]
Pittsburgh Sleep Quality Index	19-item tool that measures subjective sleep quality and disturbances Measures 7 domains: 5 related to sleep, and single domains of daytime dysfunction and medication Designed to assess sleep quality during past month Score ranges from 0–21 with a cutoff score of 5	Widely used with excellent correlation coefficient and test-retest reliability[76,77] A score >5 achieved maximum sensitivity and specificity for insomnia
Insomnia Severity Index	7-item tool that measures the patient's perception of insomnia over the past month 5 point Likert scale yielding score from 0–28; 10 being cutoff for detecting insomnia. Higher scores correlate with severity Widely used for clinical research and as a metric for treatment response	Assesses severity of both nighttime and daytime components of insomnia Shown to be brief Validity and internal consistency excellent[78] Available in several languages
Epworth Sleepiness Scale	8-item tool measuring tendency toward sleepiness Simple and rapidly administered using a 4-point Likert scale Score range 0–24; $\geq$10 suggests abnormal level of sleepiness Higher scores correlate with likelihood of more severe disorder	High correlation with MSLT results[79] Widely used in several countries[80,81] and studied in patients with comorbid conditions such as MS[82]
STOP BANG	Combination of the 4-item STOP tool and the 4-item BANG tool. STOP assesses symptoms, whereas BANG identifies physical predictors of OSA Together provide a rapid, easy screening tool for patients at risk for OSA A score $\geq$2 in the STOP portion places an individual into a high-risk category Scores of the combined STOP BANG test are reliable predictors of OSA. Probabilities for moderate/severe OSA increased from 0.36 to 0.60 as the score increased from 3 to 7 and 8	The STOP portion validity similar to the Berlin questionnaire[83] to screen for OSA A STOP BANG score of $\geq$3 has shown a high sensitivity for detecting OSA: 93% and 100% for moderate and severe OSA, respectively[84]

Berlin	10-item questionnaire covering 3 domains, including snoring, hypertension, obesity and daytime sleepiness Scoring slightly time consuming and more complicated than other instruments Developed in 1999; widely used	Sensitivity and specificity 86% and 77% respectively at a cutoff of AHI>5 and 54% and 97% for a cutoff of AHI>15.7 Validity tested in medical/surgical patients and available in several languages[83]
International Restless Leg Scale	10-item subjective tool for measuring severity of disease Domains included intensity and frequency of symptoms as well as impact on daytime function Easily administered with ordinal scoring Score of 0 = no disease Higher scores correlate with severity	Does not examine all aspects of RLS syndrome (all involved limbs and speed of onset when patient sits down) Concurrent validity with restless Legs Syndrome Quality of Life questionnaire and overall life impact score[85]
GAD-7	7-item questionnaire to assess the presence of GAD Shortened version of the GAD-13; easily administered and scored Possible score of 0–21 with a cut point of 8 to detect disease	Sensitivity and specificity 89% and 82% respectively at a cutoff of $\geq$10 Useful to detect overlap of other disorders such as PTSD, panic disorder, and SAD[86]
Beck Depression Inventory[87]	21-item questionnaire on a 4-point Likert scale used to assess the intensity of depression symptoms Measured both cognitive and somatic symptoms Shortened to an 11-item version by original investigators in 1996 (Beck) Total score range from 0–63; higher scores suggest more severe symptoms	First developed in 1961 and is one of the most frequently used instruments in adolescents, adults, and elderly Recent revisions consistent with American Psychological Association 4th ed. DSMV-IV criteria Weaker to assess other disorders such as anxiety[88]
FOSQ	The FOSQ-10 is a shortened version of the FOSQ-30 Used to measure the daytime impact of sleepiness on activities of daily living 10-item questionnaire measuring 5 factors: activity level, vigilance, sexual intimacy, and sexual relationships	Excellent validity and reliability Available in 51 languages[89] Mainstay tool in the assessment of sleep disorder clinics

Abbreviations: DSMV-IV, Diagnostic and Statistical Manual of Mental Disorders, Fourth Edition; FOSQ, Functional Outcomes of Sleep Quality; GAD, Generalized Anxiety Disorder; MS, multiple sclerosis; MSLT, multiple sleep latency testing; OSA, obstructive sleep apnea; PTSD, posttraumatic stress disorder; RLS, restless legs syndrome; SAD, seasonal affective disorder; STOP BANG, snoring, tired, observed apnea, blood pressure high, body mass index, age, neck circumference, gender.

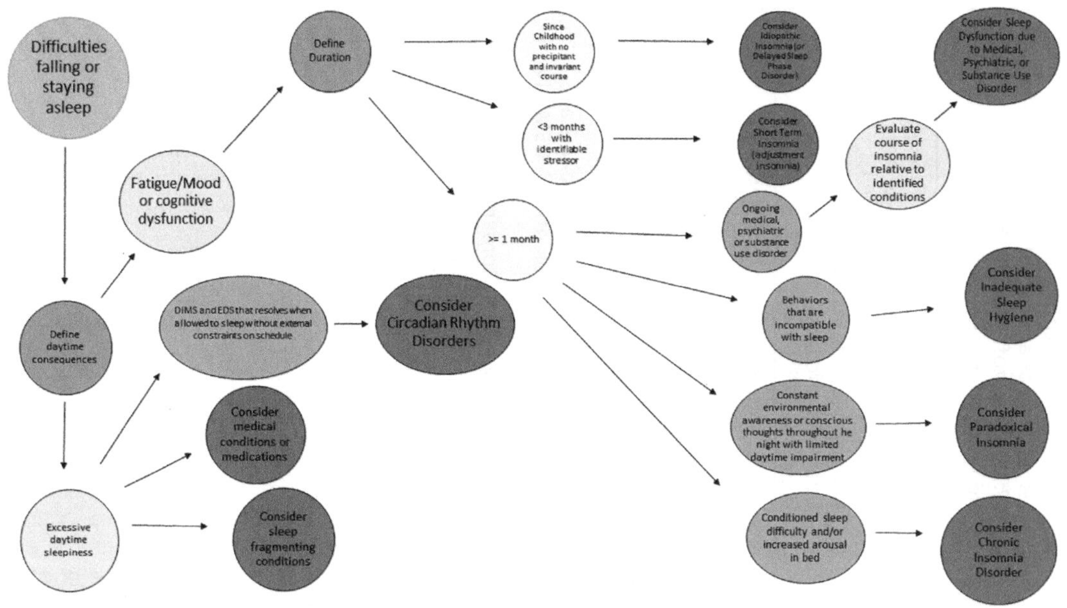

Fig. 1. Basic algorithm for the evaluation of sleep-related complaints. DIMS, difficulties initiating or maintaining sleep; EDS, excessive daytime somnolence. (*Adapted from* Arnedt JT, Conroy DA, Posner DA, et al. Evaluation of the Insomnia Patient. Clin Sleep Med 2006;1(3):319–32; and *Data from* American Academy of Sleep Medicine. International classification of sleep disorders. In: Sateia M, editor. Diagnostic and coding manual. 2nd edition. Westchester (IL): American Academy of Sleep Medicine; 2005.)

underlying cause. A patient who has difficulties falling asleep but also has complaints of difficulties waking as well as profound sleepiness during the day does not entirely fit this hyperarousal model, and may suggest a different primary condition driving these symptoms (**Figs. 2** and **3**).

Box 1
Core data points in taking a sleep history

- Bedtimes (weekday and weekend)
- Intended wake time (weekday) (with or without an alarm?)
- Wake time (weekend) (with or without an alarm?)
- Vertical wake time (weekday and weekend)
- Lights-out time (weekday and weekend)
- Sleep latency (weekday and weekend) (after lights out)
- Estimated average sleep times
- Perceived sleep quality
- Restfulness of sleep
- Degree of daytime sleepiness
- Frequency, timing, and duration of naps
- Signs and symptoms of obvious sleep disorders (for example, snoring, witnessed apneas, restless legs syndrome symptoms, leg kicking, sleep walking, dream enactment)
- Previous treatments or diagnostic testing

CIRCADIAN RHYTHM DISORDERS

To further explore these potential causes or predisposing contributions to sleep onset difficulties,

Box 2
Common sleep-prohibitive behaviors

- Exposure to electronics
- Exercise close to bedtime
- Caffeine
- Excessive napping
- Prolonged time in bed before lights out
- Television and reading in bed
- Environmental disturbances (noise, light)
- Napping
- Activating medications before bedtime
- Engaging in anxiety-provoking thoughts/activities near or at bedtime
- Evening meal close to bedtime
- Alcohol (generally affecting middle and late difficulties)
- Stimulant medications in the afternoons/evenings

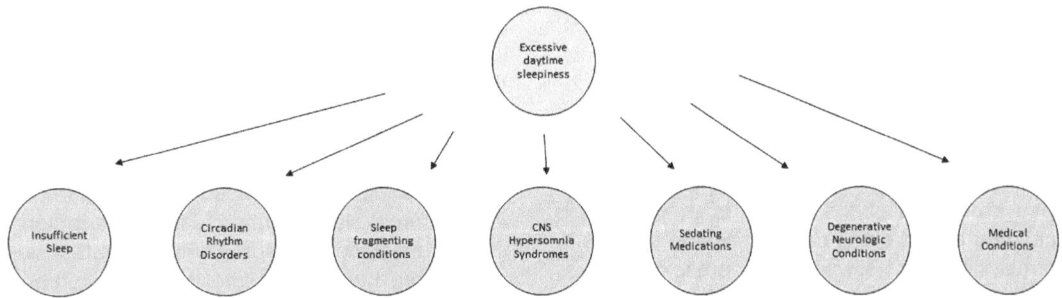

Fig. 2. Causes of excessive daytime sleepiness.

attempting to establish the chronotype of an individual can be helpful and is often essential in effectively treating patients with this complaint.

Studies have shown that a large percentage of patients with sleep onset insomnia have a delayed circadian tendency,[46] and, if characterized appropriately, a large number of patients previously labeled as having insomnia may be found to have a primary circadian rhythm disorder responsible for their symptoms. In the case of sleep onset difficulties, the circadian rhythm disorder most commonly implicated in the clinical setting is delayed sleep phase disorder (see **Fig. 3**). A clue that is often revealing is the tendency not only to have difficulties falling asleep but also to have difficulties waking in the mornings, and for patients to tend to improve or resolve when afforded the opportunity to sleep in accordance with their own schedules, such as on weekends or vacations.[47]

CLINICAL VIGNETTE

A 38-year-old woman presents to your office complaining of sleep onset difficulties. She states that she has never been able to sleep. On further questioning, she states that she is not a morning person and every night after 8 PM, gets a second wind. Her weekday bedtime is 10 PM, reading on her IPad until lights out at 11:30 PM. She is not sleepy when she goes to bed and not sleepy at lights-out time. She states that her average sleep onset latency is 60 to 90 minutes, and her sleep is light until around 4 AM when she at last feels that she is sleeping deeply. Her mandated wake time is 6 AM by alarm and she has great difficulties waking in the mornings. She has fallen asleep at traffic lights when driving to work. At weekends, her bedtime and lights-out time averages 2 AM, with a sleep latency of less than 15 minutes, and her spontaneous final wake time averages

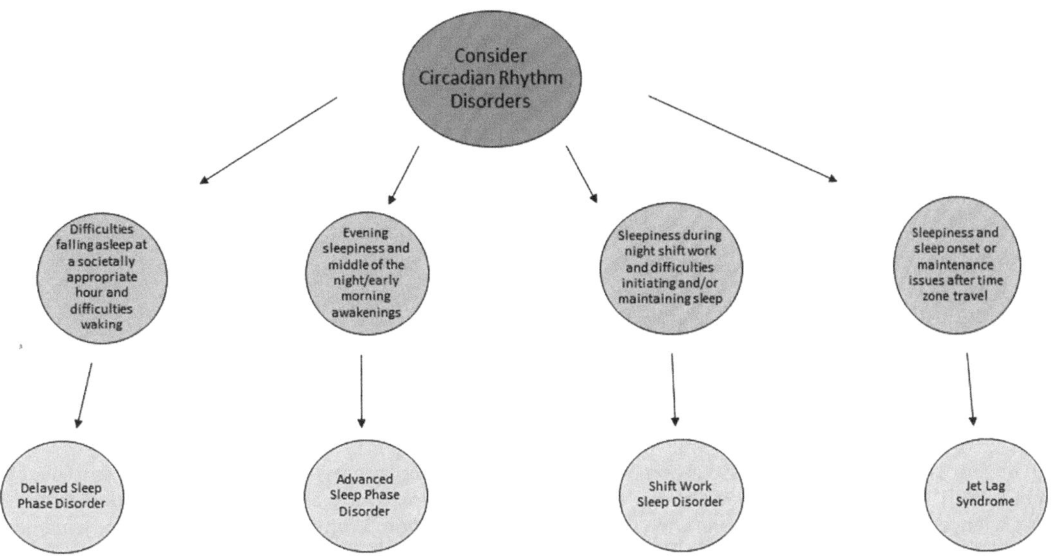

Fig. 3. Situations in which to consider circadian rhythm disorder.

around 10 AM, at which time she feels refreshed and alert.

NIGHTTIME AND EARLY MORNING AWAKENINGS

Waking during sleep is a normal component of the sleep process over the course of a night, often occurring during sleep cycle transition periods in normal sleepers. However, the presence of frequent awakenings and/or difficulties reinitiating sleep leading to prolonged wake after sleep onset is abnormal. Middle-of-the-night awakenings have several potential causes that may often be revealed through the use of preevaluation questionnaires.

The 2-Process Model and Homeostatic Load Issues

Homeostatic pressure on sleep (process S) is the biological concept that sleep drive increases with longer periods of wakefulness between intervening sleep periods. The circadian system (process C) is an opposing process that counters the accruing sleepiness as time passes by increasing the alerting signal emanating from the suprachiasmatic nucleus proportionally to the accruing sleep loss. These processes have been termed the 2-process model and are broadly thought to be how sleep and wake are regulated.[48] Sleep initiation at the beginning of the nocturnal sleep period occurs at a time when the homeostatic pressure is at its highest, and a concurrent reduction in the alerting signal allows the initial sleep onset. The first portion of the nocturnal sleep period is largely attributed to the homeostatic pressure, which creates sleep momentum that carries into the latter portion of the sleep period, at which time the reduced alerting signal allows sleep to continue until the natural circadian sleep offset time (**Fig. 4**).[49]

Homeostatic load issues are generally manifested in the form of nighttime awakenings, and often are by-product of circadian misalignment. This misalignment may not be the result of an overt circadian rhythm disorder, but rather of the well-intended individual who wants to go to bed early to get more sleep. However, if sleep onset occurs earlier than the endogenous, circadian-dependent sleep period, these two processes are unable to interact in this reciprocal manner. Nighttime awakenings subsequently tend to emerge (as well as light sleep) after the initial sleep period, which is primarily mediated by the homeostatic pressure for sleep alone. As an alternative, those individuals

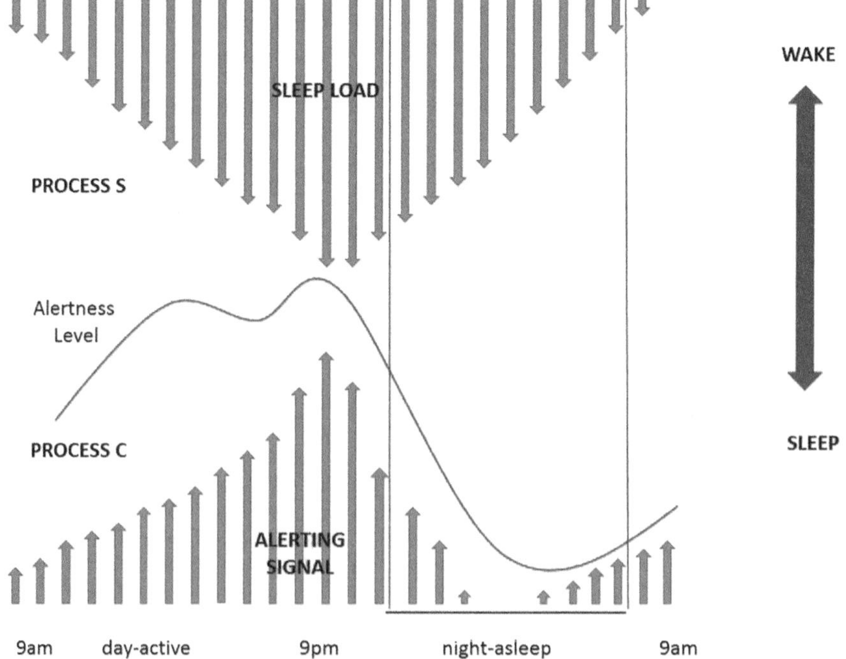

Fig. 4. The 2 process model. Process S is homeostatic pressure on sleep; process C is the circadian system. (*Adapted from* Kilduff TS, Kushida CA. Circadian regulation of sleep. In: Chokroverty S, editor. Sleep disorders medicine: basic science, technical considerations and clinical aspects. 2nd edition. Woburn (MA): Butterworth-Heinemann; 1999. p. 143; and Kennaway DJ, Voultsios A. Circadian rhythm of free melatonin in human plasma. J Clin Endocrinol Metab 1998;83(3):1013–5.)

with advanced sleep phase disorder typically present with early morning awakenings caused by their biologically determined early morning wake times.[50] Although these patients often feel sleepy in the early evening hours (suggesting a biologically mediated bedtime), they often push beyond this time because of social pressures and responsibilities, thus resulting in sleep curtailment and the appearance of early morning awakenings. Disorganization of sleep/wake periods may also predispose patients to both sleep onset difficulties and nighttime awakenings (ie, napping at inappropriate times or for excessive periods).

SLEEP-FRAGMENTING CONDITIONS

Sleep-fragmenting conditions are also a common cause of nighttime awakenings, the most common being the sleep-related breathing disorders. Beyond the sleep-fragmenting effects of these conditions, the autonomic response to a respiratory event preceding the awakening provides a fertile physiologic landscape for the alerting mechanism to be engaged. These events invite sleep-prohibitive behaviors and cognition that prolong the period before reinitiation of sleep. Periodic limb movement disorder, partial arousal conditions, nocturnal seizures, and dream enactment may also have the same effect. Nocturia, pain conditions, and environmental disturbances are also important to screen for because these conditions often contribute to these complaints as well (**Fig. 5**).

MEDICAL CONDITIONS

As mentioned previously, medical conditions and associated medications may play an important role in sleep/wake complaints. Almost any untreated or poorly controlled organ system dysfunction can cause or exacerbate sleep problems. Common conditions that may play a role in this manner include but are not limited to asthma and chronic obstructive pulmonary disease, heart failure, cardiac arrhythmias, nocturnal angina, gastroesophageal reflux disease, thyroid disease, neurologic disease (nocturnal seizures, Parkinson disease, other neuromuscular disorders), rheumatologic conditions (rheumatoid arthritis, systemic lupus erythematosus, fibromyalgia), and other pain conditions.

Miro and colleagues[51] highlighted sleep difficulties in patients with fibromyalgia. These difficulties contribute to the syndrome of fibromyalgia by inhibiting alertness and cognitive function. Increased overnight sympathetic activity has been shown to cause circadian autonomic metabolic dysfunction, which increases arousability during sleep in this population.[52] Patients with autism spectrum disorders (ASD), may present to a primary care practice with a sleep complaint. As many as 25% of parents of children diagnosed with ASD had reported their child's sleeping

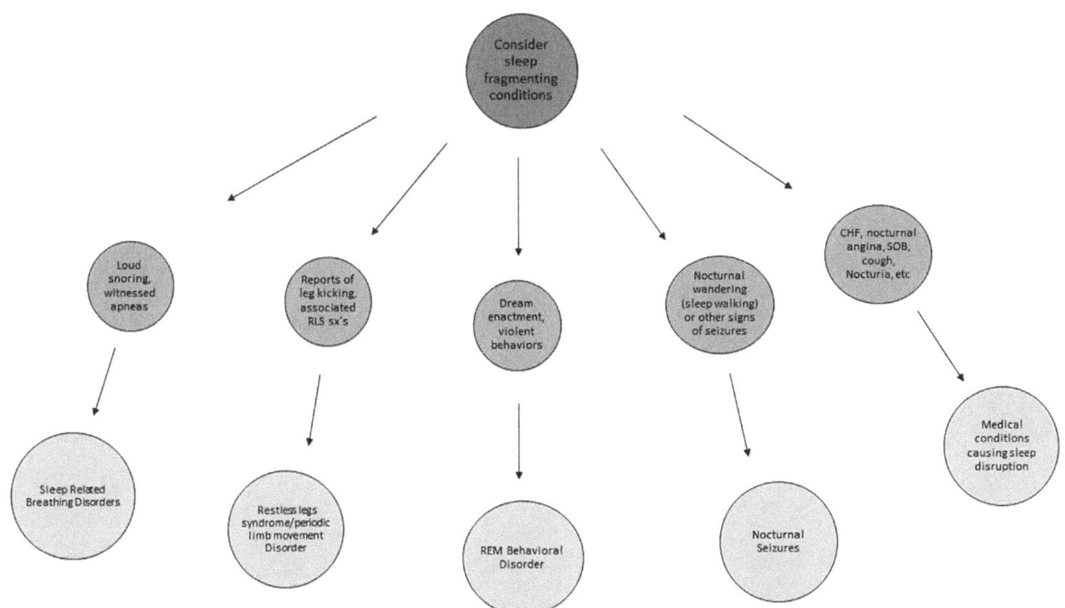

Fig. 5. Situations in which to consider sleep-fragmenting conditions. CHF, congestive heart failure; REM, rapid eye movement; RLS, restless legs syndrome; SOB, shortness of breath; sx's, symptoms.

problems. Increased awareness leads to heightened suspicion for and earlier detection of ASD in the pediatric population.[53]

Acknowledging these comorbid conditions and associated medications is often crucial in this evaluation process, and they often contribute to complaints of sleep dysfunction and/or fatigue and hypersomnolence (**Fig. 6**).

PSYCHIATRIC CONDITIONS

The complaint of insomnia, irrespective of the subtype, is a risk factor for a range of psychiatric morbidities such as substance abuse, anxiety, and suicidality.[54–56] Sleep complaints and symptoms of insomnia are present in 20% to 40% of individuals with mental illness.[6] Most (89%) patients with a dual diagnosis of substance abuse and posttraumatic stress disorder, bipolar disorder, or major depressive disorder, endorse sleep difficulties.[57] Chronic difficulty with sleep initiation has been found to precede the onset of depression, suggesting that the two conditions have a bidirectional relationship,[58] and should be considered in the differential in patients with this complaint. Severe insomnia complaints were prevalent in 25% to 46% of individuals with mood disorders or anxiety disorders compared with 12% to 24% with no disorder.[59] An eveningness chronotype has been found to be associated with depression symptom severity,[60] bipolar I disorder,[61] substance abuse,[62] and schizophrenia.[63] Nonetheless, the presence of a sleep complaint does not necessarily mean that a mental condition is present. In contrast, the mental disorder can develop as a by-product of the evolution of the underlying sleep dysfunction. Although there is a clear reciprocal relationship between psychiatric disorders and sleep, attributing sleep complaints to these underlying psychiatric conditions is often inaccurate and should not be the initial assumption when evaluating patients with these comorbidities.

DIAGNOSTIC AND ASSESSMENT TOOLS

Once a differential diagnosis list has been generated, more information and/or data should be gathered in order to better characterize the current state of the patient's complaints or to rule out potential contributors, in the same way clinicians approach the evaluation and management of any complaint.

SLEEP DIARIES

Sleep diaries are the most important and commonly used tool in the clinical setting in treating patients with sleep complaints.[32] Patients with sleep complaints tend to have recall, self-report biases when asked for retrospective recall of their sleep patterns and nightly sleep durations, and sleep diaries have been found to be less susceptible to this bias.[64] Patients ideally record their previous day/night's sleep pattern the following day, and do so on a daily basis. However, sleep diaries are not entirely reliable because patients with insomnia tend to overestimate initial sleep onset latency and time awake during the night and underestimate the total sleep time.[65] Nonetheless, sleep diaries are inexpensive and actively engage the patient in the evaluation and treatment process, further enlisting them into the collaborative endeavor of their treatment. A minimum of 2 weeks of diaries should be collected in order to effectively account for variability in sleep patterns, and up to 4 weeks is preferred.[66] Sleep diaries have a variety of formats, but should include important content

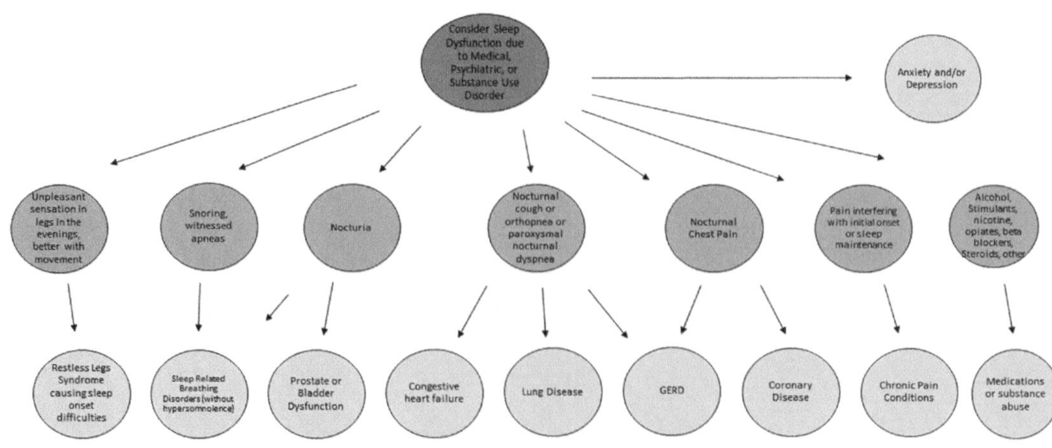

Fig. 6. Situations in which to consider sleep dysfunction caused by medical, psychiatric, or substance use disorder. GERD, gastrointestinal reflux disease.

irrespective of the format: bedtimes, lights-out time, estimated sleep onset latency, awakenings and/or time spent awake during the night, wake times, and nap times. Sleep efficiency, a calculation of time asleep divided by the total sleep time (lights-out to lights-on time) multiplied by 100 (giving a percentage of sleep time), is an important sleep parameter used to help establish a baseline and then to track treatment outcomes.[67]

ACTIGRAPHY

A more objective means of tracking sleep/wake patterns is the use of actigraphy. An actigraph is small electronic device that is typically worn around the wrist of the user's nondominant hand and that uses a piezoelectric accelerometer to track movement as a surrogate for wake and sleep. It does not measure sleep directly but correlates fairly well with sleep and wake by measuring activity.[68] Actigraphy is useful when attempting to evaluate circadian rhythm disorders and has a high degree of reliability compared with self-reported sleep diaries.[69] There are now several commercially available fitness tracking devices that use actigraphy to gather sleep and wake patterns and that have made access to this technology easier and readily available. Clinicians must be cautious when interpreting the sleep data from these devices because the technology has not been validated in patients with sleep disorders, and actigraphy has not been validated as a means with which to characterize individual stages of sleep.

SLEEP TESTING

Polysomnography (PSG) should be considered if there is concern about sleep-fragmenting conditions, parasomnias, or CNS hypersomnia syndromes. It is not indicated for the evaluation of insomnia or circadian rhythm disorders.[70] There is a potential application of PSG in evaluating circadian rhythm disorders in order to help better characterize the endogenously timed circadian phase through the layout of sleep architecture relative to the clock time; however, this indication does not meet the third-party payers' standard of medical necessity. Home sleep testing has become an accepted modality used to diagnose straightforward sleep-related breathing disorders and can be used in place of polysomnography when appropriate.[71] Multiple sleep latency testing is appropriately used in the evaluation of excessive daytime somnolence in order to diagnose and delineate CNS hypersomnia syndromes.[72] This test is not indicated to measure the perceived sleepiness or fatigue associated with insomnia. When evaluating patients for sleep-fragmenting conditions as well as CNS hypersomnia syndromes, accounting for estimated circadian delays in terms of sleep period is essential to obtain the most accurate characterization of sleep and dysfunction therein.[73]

LABORATORY TESTING AND OTHER ASSESSMENTS

Medical conditions that may be responsible or exacerbating contributors to the patient's symptoms need to be considered. Laboratory testing that should be considered when evaluating a patient with sleep/wake complaints should be based on the patient's primary complaint. For patients with both insomnia complaints and fatigue, consideration for endocrine conditions, hematologic abnormalities, renal or liver dysfunction, and/or vitamin deficiencies should be given. Thyroid function tests, a complete blood count, a complete metabolic profile, vitamin B_{12} levels, and vitamin D levels may therefore have some utility based on the clinical circumstances. The same laboratory test panel is generally applicable in patients with complaints of hypersomnolence. There are rare circumstances in which adrenal dysfunction or pituitary dysfunction may simulate similar symptoms; however, further evaluation should be based on clinical circumstances. In patients with restless legs syndrome and/or periodic limb movement disorder, low CNS iron has been clearly implicated as a cause or an exacerbating factor in this condition.[74] Serum ferritin levels correlate well with CNS iron levels and should be checked accordingly. However, there is no commercially available assay for measurement of an individual's chronotype, and the use of salivary testing for dim light melatonin onset is not practical in the clinical setting.

PSYCHOLOGICAL AND NEUROBEHAVIORAL TESTING

As previously stated, there is clearly a tight link between sleep disorders and psychiatric conditions; however, beyond screening for these types of conditions, there is little role for formal psychological assessments in the routine evaluation and management of patients with sleep/wake complaints. Patients with sleep disorders often have neurocognitive consequences; however, the use of formal neurocognitive testing is generally unnecessary unless there is concern for an evolving dementia process. In addition, symptoms of inattention and difficulties with focus and task completion are often reported in this population of patients.

Formal testing for attention deficit/hyperactivity disorder may be warranted, preferably after the sleep condition has been effectively addressed.

SUMMARY

Sleep and wake complaints generally represent a broad, complex array of potential causative disorders that must be considered in the management of these patients. The treatment approach varies drastically for the same complaint when originating from different sources. Treatment outcomes are invariably less than optimal when treatments are directed toward the symptom as opposed to the problem. A basic fund of knowledge is required by evaluating clinicians in order to interpret symptoms and generate a broad differential diagnosis list. The evaluation and management of patients with sleep and wake complaints should not be exclusively under the purview of sleep specialists, but more focused education for medical students and primary care providers is needed in order to facilitate more effective initial evaluation and management by the PCP before escalating the patient's management to the domain of the specialist. Although a validated, standardized, structured evaluation process has not been developed to date, directing care that is largely based on the standard approach used in the evaluation of any complaint should provide a reasonable basis with which to proceed with the evaluation and management process. Validation of a distilled form of the various screening and assessment tools is needed and would provide an invaluable tool for the non-BCSS clinical practice. In the coming years, an absolute need for a stronger partnership with PCPs and BCSS will be shown and further development of the bridge between the education, screening, evaluation, and management of patients with sleep and wake complaints will be mandatory.

REFERENCES

1. Institute of Medicine. Sleep disorders and sleep deprivation: an unmet public health problem. Washington, DC: The National Academies Press; 2006.
2. Ohayon MM. Prevalence of DSM-IV diagnostic criteria of insomnia: distinguishing insomnia related to mental disorders from sleep disorders. J Psychiatr Res 1997;31(3):333–46.
3. Leger D, Guilleminault C, Dreyfus JP, et al. Prevalence of insomnia in a survey of 12,778 adults in France. J Sleep Res 2000;9(1):35–42.
4. Ford DE, Kamerow DB. Epidemiologic study of sleep disturbances and psychiatric disorders. An opportunity for prevention? JAMA 1989;262(11): 1479–84.
5. Weissman MM, Greenwald S, Nino-Murcia G, et al. The morbidity of insomnia uncomplicated by psychiatric disorders. Gen Hosp Psychiatry 1997; 19(4):245–50.
6. Ohayon MM. Epidemiology of insomnia: what we know and what we still need to learn. Sleep Med Rev 2002;6(2):97–111.
7. Miles L, Dement WC. Sleep and aging. Sleep 1980; 3:119–220.
8. Young T. Rationale, design, and findings from the Wisconsin Sleep Cohort Study: toward understanding the societal burden of sleep-disordered breathing. In: Sleep Medicine Clinics, Bixler E, editors. Epidemiology of sleep disorders: clinical implications. Philadelphia: WB Saunders; 2009. p. 37–46.
9. Szentkirályi A, Madarász CZ, Novák M. Sleep disorders: impact on daytime functioning and quality of life. Expert Rev Pharmacoecon Outcomes Res 2009;9(1):49–64.
10. Fulda S, Schulz H. Cognitive dysfunction in sleep disorders. Sleep Med Rev 2001;5(6):423–45.
11. Buysse DJ, Angst J, Gamma A, et al. Prevalence, course, and comorbidity of insomnia and depression in young adults. Sleep 2008;31:473–80.
12. Pigeon WR. Insomnia as a risk factor for disease. In: Buysee DJ, Sateia MJ, editors. Insomnia: Diagnosis and treatment. New York: Informa Healthcare; 2010. p. 31–41.
13. Walsh JK, Engelhardt CL. The direct economic costs of insomnia in the United States for 1995. Sleep 1999;22(Suppl 2):S386–93.
14. Kessler R, Berglund P, Coulouvrat C, et al. Insomnia and the performance of US workers from the America Insomnia Survey. SLEEP 2011; 34(9):1161–71.
15. Somers VK, White DP, Amin R, et al. Sleep apnea and cardiovascular disease: an American Heart Association/American College of Cardiology Foundation scientific statement from the American Heart Association Council for High Blood Pressure Research Professional Education Committee, Council on Clinical Cardiology, Stroke Council, and Council on Cardiovascular Nursing in collaboration with the National Heart, Lung, and Blood institute national Center on Sleep Disorders Research (National Institutes of Health). J Am Coll Cardiol 2008;52(8):686–717.
16. Sassani A, Findley LJ, Kryger M, et al. Reducing motor vehicle collisions, costs, and fatalities by treating obstructive sleep apnea. Sleep 2004; 27(3):453–8.
17. Papp KK, Penrod CE, Strohl KP. Knowledge and attitudes of primary care physicians toward sleep and sleep disorders. Sleep Breath 2002;6:103–9.
18. Rosen RC, Rosekind M, Rosevear C, et al. Physician education in sleep and sleep disorders: a

national survey of US medical schools. Sleep 1993; 1:249–54.
19. Teodorescu MC, Avidan AY, Teodorescu M, et al. Sleep medicine content of major medical textbooks continues to be underrepresented. Sleep Med 2007;8(3):271–6.
20. Mindell JA, Bartle A, Wahab NA, et al. Sleep education in medical school curriculum: a glimpse across countries. Sleep Med 2011;12(9):928–31.
21. National Sleep Foundation. Sleep in America poll. Annapolis (MD): WB&A Market Research; 2003.
22. National Sleep Foundation. 2005 Sleep in America poll summary of findings. Washington, DC: National Sleep Foundation; 2005.
23. US Food and Drug Administration. 2013. Available at: http://www.fda.gov/drugs/drugsafety/ucm334033.htm. Accessed May 14, 2013.
24. Busto U, Sellars EM, Naranjo CA, et al. Withdrawal reaction after long term therapeutic use of benzodiazepines. N Engl J Med 1986;315:854–9.
25. Herings RM, Stricker BH, de Boer A, et al. Benzodiazepines and the risk of falling leading to femur fractures. Dosage more important than elimination half-life. Arch Intern Med 1995;55:1801–7.
26. Hemmelgarn B, Suissa S, Huang A, et al. Benzodiazepine use and the risk of motor vehicle crash in the elderly. JAMA 1997;278:27–31.
27. Salzman C, Fisher J, Nobelk Glassman R. Cognitive improvement following benzodiazepine discontinuation in elderly nursing home residents. Int J Geriatr Psychiatry 1992;7:89–93.
28. Billioti de Gage S, Bégaud B, Bazin F. Benzodiazepine use and risk of dementia: prospective population based study. BMJ 2012;345:e6231.
29. Schramm E, Hohagen F, Grasshoff U, et al. Test-retest reliability and validity of the structured interview for sleep disorders according to DSM-III-R. Am J Psychiatry 1993;150(6):867–72.
30. Ohayon MM, Guilleminault C, Zulley J, et al. Validation of the sleep-EVAL system against clinical assessments of sleep disorders and polysomnographic data. Sleep 1999;22:925–30.
31. Morin C, LeBlanc M, Daley M, et al. Epidemiology of insomnia: prevalence, self-help treatments and consultations initiated, and determinants of help-seeking behaviors. Sleep Med 2005;7(2): 123–30.
32. Sateia M, Doghramji K, Hauri P, et al. Evaluation of chronic insomnia. Sleep 2000;23(2):243–308.
33. Thornton JD, Chandriani K, Thornton J, et al. Assessing the prioritization of primary care referrals for polysomnogram. Sleep 2010;33(9):1255–60.
34. Parthasarthy S, Haynes PL, Budhiraja R. A national survey of the effect of sleep medicine specialists and American Academy of Sleep Medicine Accreditation on Management of Obstructive Sleep Apnea. J Clin Sleep Med 2006;2(2):133–42.
35. Pamidi S, Knutson KL, Ghods F, et al. The impact of sleep consultation prior to a diagnostic polysomnogram on continuous positive pressure adherence. Chest 2012;141(1):51–7.
36. Sivertsen B, Omvik S, Pallesen S, et al. Cognitive behavioral therapy vs zopiclone for treatment of chronic primary insomnia in older adults: a randomized controlled trial. JAMA 2006;296(24):2851–8.
37. Chai-Coestzer CL, Antic NA, Rowland LS, et al. Primary vs specialist sleep center management of obstructive sleep apnea and daytime sleepiness and quality of life. JAMA 2013;309(10):997–1004.
38. Krell SB, Kapur VK. Insomnia complaints in patients evaluated for obstructive sleep apnea. Sleep Breath 2005;9(3):104–10.
39. National Institutes of Health. National Institutes of Health State of the Science Conference Statement on Manifestations and Management of Chronic Insomnia is Adult, June 13-15, 2005. Sleep 2005; 28(9):1049–57.
40. Drake C, Richardson G, Roerhs T, et al. Vulnerability to stress-related sleep disturbance and hyperarousal. Sleep 2004;27(2):285–91.
41. Spielman AJ, Caruso LS, Glovinsky PB. A behavioral perspective on insomnia treatment. Psychiatr Clin North Am 1987;10(4):541–53.
42. Morin CM. Insomnia: psychological assessment and management. New York: The Guilford Press; 1993.
43. Jefferson CD, Drake CL, Scofield HM, et al. Sleep hygiene practices in a population-based sample of insomniacs. Sleep 2005;28(5):611–5.
44. Nofzinger EA, Buysse DJ, Germain A, et al. Functional neuroimaging evidence for hyperarousal in insomnia. Am J Psychiatry 2004;161(11):2126–9.
45. Stepanski E, Zorick F, Roehrs T, et al. Daytime alertness in patients with chronic insomnia compared with asymptomatic control subjects. Sleep 1988; 11(1):54–60.
46. Morris M, Lack L, Dawson D. Sleep-onset insomniacs have delayed temperature rhythms. Sleep 1990;13:1–14.
47. Regestein Q, Monk T. Delayed sleep phase syndrome: a review of its clinical aspects. Am J Psychiatry 1995;152(4):602–8.
48. Tobler I. Phylogeny of sleep regulation. In: Kryger MH, Roth T, Dement WC, editors. Principles and practices of sleep medicine. 5th edition. St Louis, Missouri: Elsevier; 2011. p. 112–3.
49. Dijk DJ, Edgar DM. Circadian and homeostatic control of wakefulness and sleep. In: Turek FW, Zee PC, editors. Regulation of sleep and circadian rhythms. New York: Marcel Dekker; 1999. p. 111–47.
50. Reid KJ, Burgess HJ. Circadian rhythm sleep disorders. Prim Care 2005;32:449–73.
51. Miro E, Lupiánez J, Hita E, et al. Attentional deficits in fibromyalgia and its relationship with pain,

emotional distress and sleep dysfunction complaints. Psychol Health 2011;26(6):765–80.
52. McMillan DE, Landis CA, Lentz MJ, et al. Heart rate variability during sleep in women with fibromyalgia. Sleep 2004;27:A724.
53. van Tongerloo MA, Bor HH. Detecting autism spectrum disorders in the general practitioner's practice. J Autism Dev Disord 2012;42:1531–8.
54. Taylor DJ, Lichstein KL, Kkurrence HH. Insomnia as a health risk factor. Behav Sleep Med 2003;1:227–47.
55. Ellis JG, Perlis ML, Bastien CH, et al. The natural history of insomnia: acute insomnia and first-onset depression. Sleep 2014;37(1):97–106.
56. Vgontzas AN, Fernandez-Mendoza JF, Bixler EO, et al. Persistent insomnia: the role of objective short sleep duration and mental health. Sleep 2012;35(1):61–8.
57. Albanese MJ, Albanese AM. Insomnia in dual diagnosis patients. Am J Addict 2010;19:382–3.
58. Yokoyama E, Kaneita Y, Saito Y, et al. Association between depression and insomnia subtypes: a longitudinal study on the elderly in Japan. Sleep 2010;33(12):1693–702.
59. Soehner AM, Harvey AG. Prevalence and functional consequences of severe insomnia symptoms in mood and anxiety disorders: results from a nationally representative sample. Sleep 2012;35(10):1367–75.
60. Drennan MD, Klauber MR, Kripke DF, et al. The effects of depression and age on the Horne-Ostberg morningness-eveningness score. J Affect Disord 1991;23:93–8.
61. Mansour HA, Wood J, Chowdari KV, et al. Circadian phase variation in bipolar I disorder. Chronobiol Int 2005;22:571–84.
62. Adan A. Chronotype and personality factors in the daily consumption of alcohol and psychostimulants. Addiction 1994;89:455–62.
63. Hofstetter JR, Mayeda AR, Happel CG, et al. Sleep and daily activity preferences in schizophrenia: associations with neurocognition and symptoms. J Nerv Ment Dis 2003;191:408–10.
64. Knab B, Engel RR. Perception of waking and sleeping: possible implications for the evaluation of insomnia. Sleep 1988;11(3):265–72.
65. Means MK, Edinger JD, Glenn DM, et al. Accuracy of sleep perceptions among insomnia sufferers and normal sleepers. Sleep Med 2003;4:285–96.
66. Lacks P, Morin CM. Recent advances in the assessment and treatment of insomnia. J Consult Clin Psychol 1992;60(4):586–94.
67. Morin CM. Measuring outcomes in randomized clinical trials of insomnia treatments. Sleep Med Rev 2003;7(3):263–79.
68. Sadeh A, Acebo C. The role of actigraphy in sleep medicine. Sleep Med Rev 2002;6:113–24.
69. Littner M, Kushida CA, Anderson WM, et al. Practice parameters for the role of actigraphy in the study of sleep and circadian rhythms: an update for 2002. Sleep 2003;26(3):337–41.
70. Littner M, Hirshkowitz M, Gramer M, et al. Practice parameters for using polysomnography to evaluate insomnia. Sleep 2003;26(6):754–60.
71. Collop NA, Anderson WM, Boehlecke B, et al. Clinical guidelines for the use of unattended portable monitors in the diagnosis of obstructive sleep apnea in adult patients. J Clin Sleep Med 2007;3(7):737–47.
72. Littner MR, Kushida C, Wise M, et al. Practice parameters for clinical use of the multiple sleep latency test and the maintenance of wakefulness test. Sleep 2005;28(1):113–21.
73. Ong JC, Huang JS, Kuo TF, et al. Characteristics of insomniacs with self-reported morning and evening chronotypes. J Clin Sleep Med 2007;3(3):289–94.
74. Earley CJ, Heckler D, Horská A, et al. The treatment of restless legs syndrome with intravenous iron dextran. Sleep Med 2004;5(3):231–5.
75. Mustafa M, Erokwu N, Ebose I, et al. Sleep problems and the risk for sleep disorders in an outpatient veteran population. Sleep Breath 2005;9:57–63.
76. Buysse DJ, Reynolds CF III, Monk TH, et al. The Pittsburgh Sleep Quality Index: a new instrument for psychiatric practice and research. Psychiatry Res 1989;28:193–213.
77. Backhaus J, Junghanns K, Brooks A, et al. Test retest reliability and validity of the Pittsburgh Sleep Quality Index in primary insomnia. J Psychosom Res 2002;53:737–40.
78. Morin C, Belleville G, Bélanger L, et al. The Insomnia Severity Index: psychometric indicators to detect insomnia cases and evaluate treatment response. Sleep 2011;34(5):601–8.
79. Johns M. Reliability and factor analysis of the Epworth Sleepiness Scale. Sleep 1992;15(4):376–81.
80. Izci B, Ardic S, Firat H, et al. Reliability and validity studies of the Turkish version of the Epworth Sleepiness Scale. Sleep Breath 2008;12(2):161–8.
81. Cho YW, Lee JH, Son HK, et al. The reliability and validity of the Korean version of the Epworth Sleepiness Scale. Sleep Breath 2011;15(3):377–84.
82. Heesen C, Nawrath L, Reich C, et al. Fatigue in multiple sclerosis: an example of cytokine mediated sickness behavior. J Neurol Neursurg Psychiatry 2006;77:34–9.
83. Chung F, Yegneswaran B, Liao P, et al. Validation of the Berlin Questionnaire and American Society of Anesthesiologists checklist as screening tools for obstructive sleep apnea in surgical patients. Anesthesiology 2008;108:288–830.
84. Chung F, Subramanyam R, Liao P, et al. High STOP-BANG score indicates a high probability of

obstructive sleep apnoea. Br J Anaesth 2012; 108(5):768–75.
85. Walters AS, LeBrocq C, Dhar A, et al. Validation of the International Restless Legs Syndrome Study Group rating scale for restless legs syndrome. The International Restless Legs Syndrome Study Group. Sleep Med 2003;4(2):121–32.
86. Spitzer RL, Kroenke K, Williams JBW, et al. A brief measure for assessing generalized anxiety disorder. Arch Intern Med 2006;166:1092–7.
87. Beck AT, Rush AJ, Shaw BF, et al. Cognitive therapy of depression. New York: Guilford Press; 1979.
88. Grothe K, Dutton G, Jones G, et al. Validation of the Beck Depression Inventory-II in a low-income African American sample of medical outpatients. Psychol Assess 2005;17(1):110–4.
89. Weaver T, Laizner A, Evans L, et al. An instrument to measure functional status outcomes for disorders of excessive sleepiness. Sleep 2010; 20(10):835–43.

Irregular Bedtimes and Awakenings

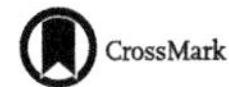

Brandon R. Peters, MD

KEYWORDS

• Irregular bedtimes • Awakenings • Circadian rhythm • Sleep disorders • Insomnia

KEY POINTS

- The body relies on a central pacemaker, the suprachiasmatic nucleus, to couple numerous physiologic patterns to the timing of light and darkness.
- Circadian rhythm disorders result when this synchrony is lost, including delayed sleep phase disorder, advanced sleep phase disorder, free-running disorder in the blind, and irregular sleep-wake disorder.
- A careful medical history with attention to symptoms of insomnia and excessive sleepiness, limited physical examination, and assessment of sleep timing with sleep logs and actigraphy may be informative.
- Treatments such as a regular sleep schedule, phototherapy, cognitive behavioral therapy for insomnia (CBTI), chronotherapy, and melatonin may be highly effective.

INTRODUCTION: NATURE OF THE PROBLEM

Like the rise and fall of the sun, sleep is presumed to be optimal when it follows a pattern of comparable regularity. Within an individual and across a population, however, there can be variability. Circadian rhythm disorders, in which patterns of wakefulness and sleep do not align with societal norms, may lead to significant problems. Lifestyle choices may also commonly affect the timing of sleep. Regardless of the cause, irregularity in the timing of sleep might compromise prompt sleep onset, introduce undesired awakenings, decrease sleep quantity and quality, and lead to important social consequences. To fully appreciate the importance of irregular sleep periods, it is necessary to have a basic understanding of the most common causes and the knowledge to evaluate and treat these disorders clinically.

Basics of Sleep and Circadian Rhythms

The propensity for sleep and wakefulness depends on 2 processes: homeostatic sleep drive and the circadian alerting system.[1] Sleep drive reflects the fact that the longer a person stays awake, the sleepier he or she will become, secondary to the buildup of chemicals within the brain that include adenosine.[2] With sleep, these natural hypnotic agents are cleared away and the desire for sleep subsides. To counteract the building sleepiness that occurs during prolonged wakefulness, the complementary circadian alerting system provides a gradually strengthened signal to stay awake.[3]

From the Latin meaning "about a day," the term circadian describes multiple endogenously generated physiologic processes that follow a nearly 24-hour pattern.[4] These processes include sleep propensity in addition to metabolism, core body

Disclosure: No relevant financial disclosures or conflicts of interest to report.

Department of Psychiatry and Behavioral Sciences, Stanford University, 100 Rowland Way, Suite 300, Novato, CA 94945, USA
E-mail address: brichp@gmail.com

Sleep Med Clin 9 (2014) 481–489
http://dx.doi.org/10.1016/j.jsmc.2014.08.001

temperature, cortisol levels, and plasma melatonin levels. These patterns rely on the interplay between elegant internal clock machinery and external time cues.

With the controls built into our genetic makeup, this machinery synchronizes rhythms that persist independently of exogenous influences. The first mammalian circadian gene, *Clock*, was identified in 1994.[5] Subsequently, multiple genes have been identified that constitute a core molecular clock that gives rise to a transcription and translation feedback loop of gene expression.[6] These genetic controls ultimately determine our body's overall circadian rhythmicity and, as a result, our risk of developing circadian rhythm disorders.

It is astounding to consider that every cell in our body follows a circadian pattern, a symphony of biochemical reactions that are perfectly timed based on available resources and orchestrated by a small group of cells in the anterior part of the brain's hypothalamus. This control center contains the master clock known as the suprachiasmatic nucleus (SCN).[7,8] Through hormonal and other as yet undetermined influences, the SCN coordinates the peripheral clocks that are present in cells as diverse as cardiac, liver, and adipose tissues.[9]

In constant conditions, the genetically determined period of biological rhythms, called tau, will be revealed.[10] It is typically more than 24 hours in length, but it may also be shorter. To realign this innate rhythmicity to synchronize with the actual geologic patterns of light and darkness, exogenous zeitgebers (from the German for "time givers") must be present.[4] This concept has important implications for the clinical treatment of the circadian rhythm sleep disorders.

Overview of the Circadian Rhythm Sleep Disorders

Disorders that are characterized by irregular bedtimes and awakenings are typically classified into several broad categories. The inability to fall or stay asleep may occur with insomnia, as discussed elsewhere. However, the most relevant disorders include those that directly affect the timing of the circadian rhythm.

How can the timing of sleep be disordered? This issue is ultimately one of perspective, influenced by social context. One must be careful in labeling normal variations of physiologic patterns such as sleep. When they lead to significant social and occupational dysfunction, however, it may be helpful to seek both diagnosis and treatment. Fortunately, for those whose irregular sleep patterns are without consequence, medical help is not typically sought.

In considering the circadian rhythm sleep disorders, it is important to understand not only the general characteristics but also the overall prevalence. These conditions are discussed in the remainder of this section and are summarized in **Box 1**.

Delayed sleep phase disorder

This condition is characterized by a delay in sleep onset and wake time by 3 to 6 hours relative to conventional sleep timing.[11] As a result, the patient will often initiate sleep between 2 and 6 AM and wake between 10 AM and 1 PM. Affected individuals often have sleep-onset insomnia, associated with increased alertness at night, and difficulty awakening at a socially acceptable time. It may be associated with prolonged hypnotic use and alcohol use at bedtime.[12] Caffeine and evening light exposure may exacerbate the condition. When sleep does occur, it is normal. It may result in impaired school and work performance, tardiness, absenteeism, and financial and relationship difficulties.

Delayed sleep phase disorder more often affects adolescents, but may persist throughout life. The prevalence among adolescents and young adults is estimated to be 7%.[13] It may drop to 0.7% among middle-aged adults.[14] Among patients presenting with complaints of insomnia to a sleep disorders clinic, up to 16% had the condition.[15] A positive family history exists in 40% of individuals.[16]

Advanced sleep phase disorder

At the other extreme, advanced sleep phase disorder is characterized by sleep and wake times that involuntarily occur 3 hours earlier than typical. Irresistible sleepiness may occur in the early evening, and early morning awakenings follow from 2 to 5 AM with complaints of insomnia. These awakenings occur even if bedtime is successfully delayed, often resulting in sleep deprivation. When sleep does occur, it is normal.[17]

The exact prevalence of advanced sleep phase disorder is unknown, but it is presumed to be rare and may not come to medical attention.[18] It is estimated to affect 1% of middle-aged adults and seems to increase with aging.[14]

Box 1
Circadian rhythm sleep disorders

Delayed sleep phase disorder

Advanced sleep phase disorder

Free-running disorder, or non–24-hour sleep-wake syndrome

Irregular sleep-wake disorder

Free-running disorder or non–24-hour sleep-wake syndrome

In the absence of effective synchronization to the natural light-dark cycle, an individual's innate circadian rhythm becomes expressed. Without constraint, this typically results in a cyclical pattern of successively delayed sleep onset and wake time.[19] The propensity for sleep and wakefulness will continually shift around the actual 24-hour clock. As a result, an affected individual attempting to observe a standard schedule will gradually experience profound daytime sleepiness, with significant nocturnal insomnia every few weeks as the misalignment unfolds.

This condition is rare in sighted people, but occurs more often among the totally blind, affecting from 50% to 73% of this population.[20,21]

Irregular sleep-wake disorder

When the circadian rhythm completely degenerates, perhaps resulting from loss of the central SCN pacemaker, irregular sleep-wake disorder may occur. This condition is typically characterized by the absence of a prolonged sleep period with multiple (often 3 or more) sleep episodes of varying lengths occurring throughout the 24-hour period. These irregular sleep bouts may be accompanied by complaints of both insomnia and excessive daytime sleepiness, depending on the time of day. The total amount of sleep that occurs is often normal.[17]

The prevalence is unknown, but it may be more common among those with neurologic disorders such as dementia, or among children with intellectual disability.[22]

Other considerations for irregular sleep

Beyond these broad categories, there are other scenarios to consider when contemplating a broader differential diagnosis. Irregular bedtimes and awakenings may simply be the manifestation of behavioral or lifestyle choices. Inadequate sleep hygiene might worsen this.[22] In addition, sleep patterns might be affected as a consequence of jet lag or shift work. These problems may occur in the context of mood dysfunction or psychiatric illness, such as in depression, seasonal affective disorder, or bipolar disorder. Irregular sleep may also be exacerbated by the use of drugs, occur secondary to a medical condition, or be worsened by institutionalization. Irregular or fragmented sleep may also occur in the setting of other sleep disorders, which is a critical differentiation to make in the clinical setting.

PATIENT HISTORY

To evaluate the conditions that contribute to irregular bedtime and awakenings, it is important to identify and differentiate between the distinct causes. Questions should seek to identify the presence of associated symptoms. As might be expected, the timing of these symptoms is of critical importance. It is also imperative to recognize other disorders that might masquerade with overlapping symptoms.

The chief complaint will guide the initial line of questioning, often related to either difficulty with insomnia or excessive daytime sleepiness, with timing as appropriate to the respective disorder. Patients with circadian rhythm disorders are often symptomatic for years before coming to medical attention. Adolescents may come for evaluation sooner because of the academic consequences of their difficulties. Without careful and complete questioning, the diagnosis can be mistaken or simply missed.

A well-designed screening questionnaire can be extremely helpful. By starting with the most relevant clinical questions and expanding as appropriate to other related topics identified by the questionnaire, the clinician's efforts can be streamlined and rewarded. Some of the elements that should be evaluated include the following.

Questions About Sleep Timing

- What time do you go to bed?
- How does your sleep schedule vary (weekdays vs weekends or work days vs days off)?
- How long does it take you to fall asleep?
- What do you do if you cannot fall asleep?
- How many times on average do you wake up in the night?
- How much time is spent awake?
- What time do you get out of bed in the morning?
- On average, how much sleep do you think you need to feel rested?

Questions to Assess Circadian Preference

- What time of day would you get up if you were entirely free to plan your day?[23]
- During the first 30 minutes of the day, how tired do you feel?
- At what time in the evening do you feel tired and, as a result, in need of sleep?
- What time do you think you reach your "feeling best" peak?
- Do you consider yourself a morning or evening type of person?

Questions to Assess Insomnia

- Does body pain wake you up at night?
- Are you a restless sleeper?
- Do you have trouble falling or staying asleep?

- Do you get too little sleep at night?
- At bedtime, do you have racing thoughts, worry, or anxiety related to falling asleep?
- Do you consider yourself a light sleeper, easily disturbed by light or noise?
- Do you wake up without an alarm?
- Do you stay in bed after you have woken up?
- Have you ever used biofeedback, meditation, guided imagery, relaxation, breathing, or other techniques to aid your sleep?

Questions to Assess Daytime Sleepiness

- Is it difficult to get out of bed because of sleepiness?
- Is your sleep unrefreshing?
- Do you feel sleepy or drowsy during the day?
- Do you feel fatigued, tired, or have low energy during the day?
- Do you take naps? How many naps and for how long?
- Do you find naps to be unrefreshing?
- Do you have problems with concentration, attention, or short-term memory?
- Have you ever fallen asleep or almost fallen asleep while driving? How many times? Did it cause an accident?

Questions to Differentiate Mood or Psychiatric Disorders

- Do you have problems with anxiety, depression, or irritability?
- Have you had any recent loss of interest, feelings of guilt, decreased energy, or appetite changes?
- Have you had any recent thoughts of hurting yourself or anyone else?

Questions to Identify Potential Consequences

- If you have a bed partner, do you disturb his or her sleep?
- Does your sleep problem interfere with daily functioning?
- Do you work graveyard, evening, late, or rotating shifts?
- Do you drive a semi-truck or fly an airplane for business or pleasure?

Further questioning may be indicated to assess for symptoms of other sleep disorders, including:

- Obstructive sleep apnea
- Restless legs syndrome
- Periodic limb movements of sleep
- Narcolepsy
- Parasomnias (sleep-related behaviors)

As would occur as part of any standard medical evaluation, it is important to elicit relevant details from the broader medical history. This approach should include a complete review of the patient's medical and surgical history, in addition to hospitalizations. All medications should be assessed, including prescription, over-the-counter, and herbal supplements, with special attention paid to agents used both now and in the past as sleeping aids. Identification of any prior known allergies may guide the selection of therapeutic agents.

Additional history should include a review of any known diagnosed sleep disorders within the family. Furthermore, a detailed social history should be obtained, to include the patient's education, occupation, and habits. In particular, the use of tobacco, alcohol, and illicit drugs may be informative. As caffeine may affect sleep, the timing of use and quantity consumed should be assessed. The timing and nature of exposure to artificial light may be revealing.

The standard 14-point review of systems may be useful to identify other general medical problems that might affect sleep timing, lead to sleep disruption, or contribute to sleepiness or fatigue. Some of the complaints that may raise the possibility of another medical or psychiatric diagnosis include:

- Pain
- Weight changes
- Anxiety/depression
- Suicidal ideation
- Hallucinations
- Confusion
- Tremor
- Hair or skin changes
- Frequent urination

A thorough history can be extremely helpful in assessing irregular bedtimes and awakenings, especially when coupled with a proper physical examination and appropriate ancillary testing.

PHYSICAL EXAMINATION

In general, there are few physical examination findings that will suggest a circadian rhythm disorder, as most of those afflicted have a completely normal examination. There are 2 exceptions to this generalization, however. Although likely evident without direct examination, blindness with the complete absence of light perception is highly suggestive of someone who is likely to have a free-running disorder.[20] Similarly, a patient with evidence of dementia or intellectual disability, especially in the context of institutionalization, is highly susceptible to an irregular sleep-wake disorder.[24] Although not requisite, a formal neurologic examination may provide additional evidence for these diagnoses.

The examination is perhaps more important in identifying other disorders that may contribute to irregular nocturnal awakenings, such as obstructive sleep apnea. In this regard, the most informative part of the evaluation is careful inspection of the nasal passage, oropharynx, and craniofacial structures. Further assessment of the cardiovascular system, including identification of peripheral edema, should also routinely occur.[25]

Beyond the standard evaluation to assess risk factors for sleep apnea, the physical examination is not generally revealing. As a result, further ancillary testing may prove necessary to elucidate the condition.

SLEEP TESTS AND ADDITIONAL TESTING

Fortunately, low-tech and inexpensive assessment tools (summarized in **Box 2**) can be very helpful in identifying irregular patterns of sleep and wakefulness. Further testing can be ordered judiciously to aid diagnosis when the condition is complicated by suspected comorbid sleep disorders.

Epworth Sleepiness Scale

Perhaps the most commonly used instrument in the sleep specialist's office, the Epworth Sleepiness Scale can be helpful in identifying excessive daytime sleepiness.[26] If this sleepiness has a strongly temporal pattern, this could be useful to differentiate a circadian cause from that attributable to other sleep disorders.

Box 2
Tools for assessment of circadian rhythm sleep disorders

- Epworth Sleepiness Scale
- Sleep log
- Actigraphy
- Polysomnography
- Multiple sleep latency testing
- Maintenance of wakefulness testing
- Laboratory studies
  - Thyroid-stimulating hormone
  - Serum or urine drug screen

Sleep Log

To assess the long-term pattern of irregular bedtimes and awakenings, it is necessary to track this information over at least 7 days.[17] To accomplish this assessment, a sleep log can record basic information. This log typically will include bedtimes, wake times, total sleep time, and naps. As it relies on the recollection of and accurate reporting by the patient, more objective tracking may be needed.

Actigraphy

Actigraphy is another option for recording sleep-wake patterns over a period of weeks.[27] About the size of a wristwatch, the device measures movement with an accelerometer. It is typically worn on the nondominant arm, but can also be placed on an ankle. The associated software produces reports that can be edited to further corroborate sleep logs. The differentiation between long periods of inactivity, consistent with sleep, and periods of increased movement can identify basic sleep patterns and total sleep time. These data can be helpful in establishing a baseline, especially if formal polysomnographic studies are pursued.

Polysomnography

Though not requisite to evaluate most circadian rhythm disorders, further sleep studies may be arranged to rule out other potential causes of excessive sleepiness or insomnia such as sleep apnea or parasomnias.[17] The attended diagnostic polysomnogram remains the gold standard for evaluation of sleep disorders.

Multiple Sleep Latency Testing and Maintenance of Wakefulness Testing

Beyond the polysomnogram, studies to assess excessive sleepiness include multiple sleep latency testing and maintenance of wakefulness testing. These tests are not indicated for routine clinical assessment of insomnia or circadian rhythm disorders.[28]

Other Laboratory Studies and Imaging

Further ancillary laboratory testing may be infrequently used to rule out other potential causes of the complaints. These tests might include thyroid-stimulating hormone or a serum or urine drug screen to identify potential intoxicants.

There is currently no role for radiographic imaging in the diagnosis of irregular bedtimes and awakenings.

TREATMENT OPTIONS

With the circadian rhythm disorders there are several effective therapies that can be used. Strict adherence to the interventions is necessary to avoid a relapse of the condition. Some of the potential treatment options are discussed in this section and are summarized in **Box 3**.

Regular Sleep Schedule

It is recommended that patients with circadian rhythm disorders observe a very regular sleep schedule. Bedtime and wake time should be consistent every day, including weekends. The designated sleep epochs should be sufficient to avoid the effects of sleep deprivation.[29]

Phototherapy

Phototherapy is another commonly used treatment. Exposure to light at the proper times helps to align the circadian alerting signal.[30] For the treatment of delayed sleep phase syndrome, exposure to bright light should occur on awakening. Conversely, patients with advanced sleep phase syndrome may respond to light exposure timed to occur at night.[27]

What is the best modality to administer this light therapy? Direct sunlight is preferred, with an intensity that exceeds 100,000 lux (lux is a measure of light intensity, as defined by 1 lumen spread over 1 m^2 of area). Commercially available light boxes often have a strength of 10,000 lux. Ordinary overhead indoor office lighting may be just 500 lux.[31]

It is recommended that patients with delayed sleep phase syndrome get 30 minutes of sunlight exposure within 15 minutes of waking. If waking before dawn, this exposure can occur with the sunrise. By taking a walk, sitting outside, or engaging in other outdoor activities, the desired sunlight exposure can be obtained.

Incidental exposure of the eyes is sufficient; staring at the sun should be avoided. It is necessary to remove any hats, visors, or sunglasses that would interfere with the light encountering the eyes. Morning sunlight is relatively weak compared with that which occurs at midday, but sunscreen can be applied to the face and exposed skin if concern exists for the potential risks.

Many patients will ask if they should still go outside for sunlight exposure on days when it is overcast with clouds or raining. Although the intensity of the light is significantly diminished, it is best to reinforce the consistency of the behavior by continuing the practice on days with inclement weather.

It is important that the timing of the light exposure be appropriate. This timing varies by condition, as already indicated. Ill-timed exposure may actually shift the sleep phase in an undesired direction. For example, light exposure in the evening may cause a delayed sleep phase to become delayed even further.[32] For this reason, sensitive individuals may wish to avoid exposure to artificial light at certain times.

There is a tipping point during the night that can cause an individual to shift to one direction or to another. The overall phase can be determined by the dim-light melatonin onset.[33,34] Light exposure before this tipping point shifts the sleep phase later, whereas exposure after it shifts the phase earlier.[35] In most individuals, this tipping point occurs 2 to 3 hours before the natural awakening.

This consideration is important with significantly shifted sleep periods. Waking a person to get sunlight exposure at 7:30 AM, when they have been consistently sleeping in until 11 AM, may have adverse effects. The light may actually shift their sleep phase even later.[29] Therefore, it is best to gradually institute the changes in the sleep schedule and accompanying light exposure.

Box 3
Potential treatment options for circadian rhythm sleep disorders

- Regular sleep schedule
- Phototherapy
- Cognitive behavioral therapy for insomnia
- Chronotherapy
- Melatonin
- Further treatments
  - Prescription medications, including sleeping pills and stimulants; signals such as the timing of social activities, exercise, meals, and environmental temperature

Cognitive Behavioral Therapy for Insomnia

Many patients require support as they make these alterations. As they are working against the timing dictated by their innate circadian rhythm, lapses in adhering to the schedule will result in setbacks, which can be frustrating and undermine compliance. As a result, it can be helpful to initiate the changes as part of a structured cognitive behavioral therapy for insomnia (CBTI) program.[36]

Typically administered by a psychologist or specially trained sleep specialist, CBTI is a program of 4 to 6 weekly visits that includes sleep education and targeted changes. With the use of sleep logs, alterations and adherence can be tracked over the treatment course. By simultaneously addressing the thoughts and emotions linked to the sleep patterns, often exacerbated by social pressures, effective behavioral modification can occur. As part of the treatment, interventions such as sleep consolidation, stimulus control, and relaxation techniques can be used.[37] By teaching the patient a set of skills, relapses can be successfully maneuvered independently. If access to a CBTI specialist is problematic, online programs and workbooks also exist, although these may require more self-sufficiency and motivation on the part of the patient.

Chronotherapy

In rare cases, it may be necessary to use chronotherapy to realign a circadian rhythm, especially among those with delayed sleep phase syndrome who have difficulty initiating sleep.[12] Chronotherapy is based on an incremental delay in the sleep period by several hours over successive days until the desired sleep timing is achieved. For example, someone with delayed sleep phase syndrome who is going to sleep consistently at 3 AM but desires to go to bed at 11 PM may follow this schedule:

- Day 1: Bedtime 6 AM
- Day 2: Bedtime 9 AM
- Day 3: Bedtime 12 noon
- Day 4: Bedtime 3 PM
- Day 5: Bedtime 6 PM
- Day 6: Bedtime 9 PM
- Day 7 and thereafter: Bedtime 11 PM

This intensive treatment can be difficult to carry out at home and is sometimes done within a hospital setting. Light exposure at the wrong times may complicate the intervention. In some cases, it may be necessary to make adjustments in smaller intervals, adjusting the bedtime by only 1 or 2 hours. Once the full adjustment is accomplished, the new sleep-wake schedule must be strictly enforced to prevent relapse.

Melatonin

Melatonin can be used as an external signal to cue the timing of the circadian system.[38] Melatonin's effects are relatively weaker among the sighted, but it can be used to entrain blind patients to a normal circadian rhythm.[39] The dose and timing of administration for circadian problems also differs from its use as a hypnotic agent.

To treat delayed sleep phase syndrome, for instance, a low dose of melatonin may be taken 5 to 6 hours before the habitual bedtime. The lowest effective dose for an individual may be relatively small, perhaps less than 1 mg.[40] Higher doses may have unwanted effects, exceeding physiologic levels and resulting in residual morning effects.

Because of its mild sedative effects, it is not recommended for melatonin to be taken in the morning to treat advanced sleep phase syndrome. Instead, properly timed light exposure is preferred.[24]

Tasimelteon, sold under the brand name Hetlioz, is a melatonin agonist that is now available for the treatment of free-running disorder among the blind.[41]

Further Treatments

Prescription medications, including sleeping pills and stimulants, may be effective for the relief of symptoms of insomnia or excessive daytime sleepiness. Other signals such as the timing of social activities, exercise, meals, and environmental temperature may also influence circadian patterns.[42–44]

SUMMARY

The body relies on a central pacemaker, the suprachiasmatic nucleus, to couple numerous physiologic patterns to the timing of light and darkness. Principal among these is the circadian alerting signal and resulting pattern of sleep and wakefulness, with significant consequences when the system is unmoored from external influences. Circadian rhythm disorders may result, including delayed sleep phase disorder, advanced sleep phase disorder, free-running disorder in the blind, and irregular sleep-wake disorder. Lifestyle choice, psychiatric conditions, and substance use may also lead to irregular bedtimes and awakenings. A careful history can characterize the nature of the problem, with attention paid to the timing of symptoms of insomnia and excessive sleepiness. The physical examination may identify signs of other sleep disorders, such as sleep apnea, but may be normal in both delayed and advanced sleep phase disorders. Further assessment may require the use of sleep logs, actigraphy, and, in select cases, formal testing with polysomnography. Treatments can be highly effective and may include a regular sleep schedule, phototherapy, CBTI, chronotherapy, melatonin, and other options. These disorders can have significant psychosocial consequences, and it can be gratifying to properly identify the underlying cause and provide timely and effective intervention.

REFERENCES

1. Borbely AA. A two process model of sleep regulation. Hum Neurobiol 1982;1:195–204.
2. Porkka-Heiskanen T, Strecker RE, McCarley RW. Brain site-specificity of extracellular adenosine concentration changes during sleep deprivation and spontaneous sleep: an in vivo microdialysis study. Neuroscience 2000;99:507–17.
3. Roehrs T, Carskadon MA, Dement WC, et al. Daytime sleepiness and alertness. In: Kryger MH, Roth T, Dement WC, editors. Principles and practices of sleep medicine. St Louis (MO): Elsevier Saunders; 2011. p. 48–9.
4. Moore-Ede MC, Sulzman FM, Fuller CA. A physiological system measuring time. In: Moore-Ede MC, Sulzman FM, Fuller CA, editors. The clocks that time us. Cambridge (MA): Harvard University Press; 1984. p. 1–112.
5. Vitaterna MH, King DP, Chang AM, et al. Mutagenesis and mapping of a mouse gene, clock, essential for circadian behavior. Science 1994;264(5159):719–25.
6. Lowrey PL, Takahashi JS. Mammalian circadian biology: elucidating genome-wide levels of temporal association. Annu Rev Genomics Hum Genet 2004; 5:407–41.
7. Moore RY, Eichler VB. Loss of a circadian adrenal corticosterone rhythm following suprachiasmatic lesions in the rat. Brain Res 1972;42(1):201–6.
8. Stephan FK, Zucker I. Circadian rhythms in drinking behavior and locomotor activity of rats are eliminated by hypothalamic lesions. Proc Natl Acad Sci U S A 1972;69(6):1583–6.
9. Ramsey KM, Bass J. Animal models for disorders of chronobiology: cell and tissue. In: Kryger MH, Roth T, Dement WC, editors. Principles and practices of sleep medicine. St Louis (MO): Elsevier Saunders; 2011. p. 463–7.
10. Kleitman N. Sleep and wakefulness. Chicago: University of Chicago Press; 1963.
11. Weitzman ED, Czeisler CA, Coleman RM, et al. Delayed sleep phase syndrome: a chronobiological disorder with sleep-onset insomnia. Arch Gen Psychiatry 1981;38:737–46.
12. Czeisler CA, Richardson GS, Coleman RM, et al. Chronotherapy: resetting the circadian clocks of patients with delayed sleep phase insomnia. Sleep 1981;4:1–21.
13. Pelayo RP, Thorpy MJ, Glovinsky P. Prevalence of delayed sleep phase syndrome among adolescents. J Sleep Res 1988;17:392.
14. Ando K, Kripke DF, Ancoli-Israel S. Estimated prevalence of delayed and advanced sleep phase syndromes. Sleep Res 1995;24:509.
15. Regestein QR, Monk TH. Delayed sleep phase syndrome: a review of its clinical aspects. Am J Psychiatry 1995;152:602–8.
16. Ancoli-Israel S, Schnierow B, Kelsoe J, et al. A pedigree of one family with delayed sleep phase syndrome. Chronobiol Int 2001;18:831–41.
17. Reid KJ, Zee PC. Circadian disorders of the sleep-wake cycle. In: Kryger MH, Roth T, Dement WC, editors. Principles and practices of sleep medicine. St Louis (MO): Elsevier Saunders; 2011. p. 470–82.
18. Schrader H, Bovim G, Sand T. The prevalence of delayed and advanced sleep phase syndromes. J Sleep Res 1993;2:51–5.
19. Sack RL, Lewy AJ. Circadian rhythm sleep disorders: lessons from the blind. Sleep Med Rev 2001; 5(3):189–206.
20. Sack RL, Lewy AJ, Blood ML, et al. Circadian rhythm abnormalities in totally blind people: incidence and clinical significance. J Clin Endocrinol Metab 1992; 75:127–34.
21. Czeisler CA, Shanahan TL, Klerman EB, et al. Suppression of melatonin secretion in some blind patients by exposure to bright light. N Engl J Med 1995;332:6–11.
22. American Sleep Disorders Association. The international classification of sleep disorders: diagnostic and coding manual. 2nd edition. Westchester (IL): American Academy of Sleep Medicine; 2005.
23. Horne JA, Ostberg O. A self-assessment questionnaire to determine morningness-eveningness in human circadian rhythms. Int J Chronobiol 1976;4:97–110.
24. Sack RL, Auckley D, Auger RR, et al. Circadian rhythm sleep disorders: part II, advanced sleep phase disorder, delayed sleep phase disorder, free-running disorder, and irregular sleep-wake rhythm. An American Academy of Sleep Medicine review. Sleep 2007;20:1484–501.
25. Cao MT, Guilleminault C, Kushida CA. Clinical features and evaluation of obstructive sleep apnea and upper airway resistance syndrome. In: Kryger MH, Roth T, Dement WC, editors. Principles and practices of sleep medicine. St Louis (MO): Elsevier Saunders; 2011. p. 1213–5.
26. Johns MW. A new method for measuring daytime sleepiness: the Epworth Sleepiness Scale. Sleep 1991;14:540–5.
27. Morgenthaler T, Alessi C, Friedman L, et al. Practice parameters for the use of actigraphy in the assessment of sleep and sleep disorders: an update for 2007. Sleep 2007;30(4):519–29.
28. Standards of Practice Committee of the American Academy of Sleep Medicine. Practice parameters for clinical use of the multiple sleep latency test and the maintenance of wakefulness test. Sleep 2005;28:113–21.
29. Richardson G, Malin HV. Circadian rhythm sleep disorders: pathophysiology and treatment. J Clin Neurophysiol 1996;13:17–31.
30. Lewy AJ, Sack RL, Singer CM. Treating phase typed chronobiologic sleep and mood disorders using

appropriately timed bring artificial light. Psychopharmacol Bull 1985;21:368–72.
31. Schlyter P. Radiometry and photometry in astronomy. 2006. Available at: http://stjarnhimlen.se/comp/radfaq.html#10. Accessed: September 6, 2014.
32. Zeitzer JM, Dijk DJ, Kronauer RE, et al. Sensitivity of the human circadian pacemaker to nocturnal light: melatonin phase resetting and suppression. J Physiol 2000;526:695–702.
33. Shibui K, Uchiyama M, Okawa M. Melatonin rhythms in delayed sleep phase syndrome. J Biol Rhythms 1999;14:72–6.
34. Lewy AJ. The dim light melatonin onset, melatonin assays and biological rhythm research in humans. Biol Signals Recept 1999;8:79–83.
35. Czeisler CA, Allan JS, Strogatz SH, et al. Bright light resets the human circadian pacemaker independent of the timing of the sleep-wake cycle. Science 1986; 233:667–71.
36. Morin CM, Bootzin RR, Buysse DJ, et al. Psychological and behavioral treatment of insomnia: an update of recent evidence (1998–2004). Sleep 2006;29: 1398–414.
37. Perlis ML, Jungquist C, Smith MT. Cognitive behavioral treatment of insomnia: a session-by-session guide. New York: Springer Verlag; 2005.
38. Lewy AJ, Ahmed S, Sack RL. Phase shifting the human circadian clock using melatonin. Behav Brain Res 1996;73:131–4.
39. Sack RL, Brandes RW, Kendall AR, et al. Entrainment of free-running circadian rhythms by melatonin in blind people. N Engl J Med 2000;343(15): 1070–7.
40. Mundey K, Benloucif S, Harsanyi K, et al. Phase-dependent treatment of delayed sleep phase syndrome with melatonin. Sleep 2005;28:1271–8.
41. Hardeland R. Tasimelteon, a melatonin agonist for the treatment of insomnia and circadian rhythm sleep disorders. Curr Opin Investig Drugs 2009;10(7): 691–701.
42. Aschoff J, Fatranská M, Giedke H, et al. Human circadian rhythms in continuous darkness: entrainment by social cues. Science 1971;171: 213–5.
43. Honma K, Honma S, Nakamura K, et al. Differential effects of bright light and social cues on reentrainment of human circadian rhythms. Am J Physiol 1995;268:R528–35.
44. Buxton OM, Frank SA, L'Hermite-Balériaux M, et al. Roles of intensity and duration of nocturnal exercise in causing phase delays of human circadian rhythms. Am J Physiol 1997;273:E536–42.

Daytime Sleepiness

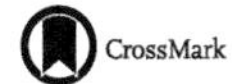

Mitchell G. Miglis, MD[a,b,*], Clete A. Kushida, MD, PhD[c]

KEYWORDS

• Sleepiness • Fatigue • Hypersomnia • Circadian rhythm disorder • Narcolepsy
• Restless leg syndrome • Obstructive sleep apnea

KEY POINTS

- Excessive daytime sleepiness is one of the most common indications for referral to the sleep clinic.
- The differential diagnosis for any patient with excessive daytime sleepiness is broad and includes primary sleep disorders, medical conditions, and mood disorders.
- Patient safety is paramount in the evaluation of any patient with excessive daytime sleepiness, and the risk of drowsy driving should always be assessed.
- Diagnosis is made primarily based on clinical history.
- Adjunctive testing such as serology, actigraphy, polysomnography, the multiple sleep latency test, and the maintenance of wakefulness test may be useful in select cases.

INTRODUCTION

Sleepiness is an extremely common symptom in our society, affecting an estimated 10% to 25% of the general population.[1] Sleepiness as a symptom is sometimes difficult for patients to describe, and 2 individuals with identical sleep patterns may report very different symptoms. The American Academy of Sleep Medicine defines excessive daytime sleepiness (EDS) as the inability to maintain wakefulness and alertness during the major waking episodes of the day, with sleep occurring unintentionally or at inappropriate times almost daily for at least 3 months.[2] EDS is a major source of vehicular accidents and loss of productivity in the workplace, and it is one of the most common indications for referral to the sleep clinic.

PATIENT HISTORY

A comprehensive sleep history is the most important aspect in the evaluation of any patient with EDS. Whenever possible, this information should be given in the company of the patient's bed partner, who may be able to provide additional history of which the patient is unaware. The Epworth Sleepiness Scale is the most commonly used validated subjective assessment of a patient's sleepiness over the last several months.[3] A score of 10 or greater typically indicates EDS.

Patients may use varying terms to describe their symptoms, which may or may not include the word *sleepiness*. Almost all of the primary sleep disorders can cause EDS (**Box 1**), however the first challenge for the clinician is to distinguish symptoms of sleepiness from those of fatigue. In many

The authors have nothing to disclose.
[a] Sleep Medicine, Neurology, Stanford University, Palo Alto, CA, USA; [b] Department of Neurology, Stanford Sleep Medicine Center, 450 Broadway Street, M/C 5704, Redwood City, CA 94063, USA; [c] Department of Psychiatry, Stanford Sleep Medicine Center, 450 Broadway Street, M/C 5704, Redwood City, CA 94063, USA
* Corresponding author. Department of Neurology, Stanford Sleep Medicine Center, Redwood City, CA.
E-mail address: mmiglis@stanford.edu

Sleep Med Clin 9 (2014) 491–498
http://dx.doi.org/10.1016/j.jsmc.2014.08.007

Box 1
Sleep disorders associated with excessive daytime sleepiness

Insufficient sleep time

Insomnia

Obstructive sleep apnea

Circadian rhythm disorders

- Delayed sleep phase syndrome
- Advanced sleep phase syndrome
- Irregular sleep phase syndrome
- Non–24-hour sleep phase syndrome
- Shift work disorder
- Jet lag disorder

Restless legs syndrome

Periodic limb movement disorder

Hypersomnias of central origin

- Narcolepsy
- Kleine-Levin syndrome
- Menstruation-related hypersomnia
- Idiopathic hypersomnia

cases, fatigue is described as body tiredness, lack of energy, or a general sense of exhaustion, whereas sleepiness is the inability to avoid falling asleep.[4]

A sleepy patient's symptoms are usually exacerbated by rest, whereas a fatigued patient's symptoms are typically exacerbated by activity. When given the opportunity to sleep, a fatigued patient may have difficulty doing so, whereas a sleepy patient will usually have no problem and often falls asleep inadvertently, as in office waiting rooms. The exception to this is the patient with insomnia, who, despite experiencing EDS or fatigue, has great difficulty falling asleep, often due to a sensation of generalized hyperarousal.

Fatigue can result from several medical and psychiatric diagnoses, and it is important to rule out primary mood disorder and general medical conditions such as anemia, hypothyroidism, renal insufficiency, and other metabolic disorders (**Box 2**). The patient's medication list should be reviewed, as there are many common medications that can contribute to EDS (**Box 3**). Activating medications should be taken in the morning when possible, and sedating medications avoided until the evening hours.

Several neurologic conditions can contribute to EDS, either as part of the primary disease process or owing to the medications used to treat the disease (**Box 4**). Although narcolepsy and restless legs syndrome (RLS) are neurologic sleep disorders, they are commonly classified as primary sleep disorders and as such are included in **Box 1**.

Some patients who describe what most clinicians would interpret as fatigue do in fact have EDS, which is evidenced by the fact that when their underlying sleep disorder is treated, their symptoms of fatigue can improve.[5]

In severe cases, EDS may lead to "sleep attacks," in which patients can suddenly and inadvertently fall asleep in active situations such as eating, talking, or driving. Patient safety is thus paramount when evaluating a patient with EDS, and the risk of drowsy driving should always be addressed during the initial visit.

In addition to the desire for sleep, patients with EDS may complain of difficulties with memory and concentration, a sensation of "brain fog," or feelings of derealization. They may also experience mood changes, such as depression, irritability, or

Box 2
Typical medical and psychiatric conditions associated with excessive daytime sleepiness and fatigue

Anemia

Hypothyroidism

End-stage renal disease

Hepatic encephalopathy

Obesity

Adrenal insufficiency

Depression

Anxiety

Substance abuse

Box 3
Medications associated with excessive daytime sleepiness

Benzodiazepines

Barbiturates

Opioid analgesics

Benzodiazepine receptor agonists

Antihistamines

Antidepressants

Antipsychotics

β-blockers

Dopaminergic medications

Box 4
Neurologic conditions associated with excessive daytime sleepiness

α synucleinopathies

- Parkinson's disease
- Dementia with Lewy bodies
- Multiple system atrophy
- Pure autonomic failure

Disorders of orthostatic intolerance

- Neurogenic orthostatic hypotension
- Postural tachycardia syndrome

Amyotrophic lateral sclerosis

Myotonic dystrophy

Traumatic brain injury

Hypothalamic structural lesions

Niemann-Pick type C

Prader-Willi syndrome

Fragile X

hyperactivity. This later symptom is especially common in children with EDS.

To help the narrow the differential, the clinician should attempt to characterize the patient's typical sleep and wake schedule. This schedule includes what time they get into bed, how long it takes them to fall asleep, what time they wake in the morning, and how frequently they wake throughout the night. If they experience frequent awakenings, is it difficult for them to fall back sleep? Do they nap during the day, either intentionally or inadvertently? The quantity and timing of caffeine consumption should be addressed. Sleep diaries are a useful tool and can be downloaded from several online sources, including the American Academy of Sleep Medicine Web site (http://yoursleep.aasmnet.org/pdf/sleepdiary.pdf). Actigraphy, which relies on a small recorder typically worn on the wrist, measures body activity to estimate sleep-wake patterns, and may be useful in the assessment of a patient's sleep-wake schedule.[6]

Key components of the sleep history in the evaluation of a patient with EDS are summarized in **Box 5**.

Insufficient Sleep Time

Insufficient sleep time is one of the most common causes of EDS in our society, and the impact of this should not be underestimated. EDS secondary to insufficient sleep time can be either self-imposed or work related, as in the circadian rhythm disorders of shift workers.

Box 5
Key components of the sleep history in the evaluation of a patient with excessive daytime sleepiness

Time in bed

Description of bedroom environment

Activities before bedtime

Sleep onset latency

Number and duration of nocturnal awakenings

Nap timing and duration

Patient's perceptions of what constitutes insufficient sleep time can vary and may be quite different from the perception of the clinician. Although each individual's sleep needs are unique and likely genetically influenced, most individuals require at least 6 hours of uninterrupted sleep to feel rested the following day. Insufficient sleep time should be considered in patients who sleep in on weekends, especially if this "catch-up sleep" extends their nightly sleep period by several hours or more.

Insomnia

Like insufficient sleep time, insomnia is extremely common, and in many ways is exacerbated by our technologically driven society. Prevalence estimates range from 6% to 18% of the general population.[7] Insomnia is defined by the International Classification of Sleep Disorders, Third Edition as difficulty initiating or maintaining sleep, early morning awakening, or nonrestorative or nonrefreshing sleep, in conjunction with daytime impairment.[2] It should be noted that daytime impairment can include either sleepiness or fatigue.

Patients with insomnia will describe difficulty falling asleep, staying asleep, or awakening earlier than anticipated in the morning. They may also describe sleep time that is sufficient, however, nonrestorative in quality. These symptoms are present despite the opportunity for adequate sleep times.

The prevalence of insomnia increases with age because of a reduction in the percentage of stage N3 non–rapid eye movement (NREM) sleep, an increase in the percentage of stages N1 and N2 NREM sleep, reduced sleep efficiency, and a reduction in the arousal threshold.

The International Classification of Sleep Disorders, Third Edition no longer uses the subtypes of psychophysiological, paradoxic, or idiopathic insomnia. Instead, patients are now divided into "chronic," with symptoms present for at least 3 months, and "short-term," with symptoms present less than 3 months. Symptoms of daytime impairment must be present at least 3 days out of the week for both subtypes.

Insomnia is a clinical diagnosis and does not require a polysomnography (PSG). Sleep diaries and actigraphy may be helpful in further characterizing a patient's sleep schedule and can aid in treatment approaches.

Circadian Rhythm Disorders

Circadian rhythm disorders can masquerade as insomnia, and these patients may also describe difficulty falling asleep, staying asleep, or awakening earlier than anticipated. This group of disorders includes those of delayed sleep-wake phase disorder (DSWPD), advanced sleep-wake phase disorder (ASWPD), irregular sleep-wake phase disorder (ISWPD), non–24-hour sleep phase disorder (Non-24), shift work disorder, and jet lag disorder. Like insomnia, patients with circadian rhythm disorders must also note symptoms of daytime impairment.

- DSWPD patients have difficulty falling asleep and difficulty awakening in the morning. Their symptoms are exacerbated on days that they have to wake up early for school or work. DSWPD is more common in adolescents and young adults.
- ASWPD patients, however, fall asleep early in the evening and awaken earlier than they would like. This condition is more common in the elderly.
- ISWPD patients do not have a clearly defined sleep or wake time. As a result, there is no clear rhythmicity to their sleep schedule. This condition is common in patients with dementing illnesses such as Alzheimer's dementia, especially in those who are institutionalized or hospitalized for prolonged periods. These environments tend to lack the reinforcement of natural circadian *zeitgeibers*, or timegivers such as light, exercise, and social interaction, further exacerbating the ISWPD in these patients.
- Non-24, or free-running type, is a circadian rhythm disorder in which an individual's sleep time gradually shifts later and later, and can eventually drift into the daytime hours. This condition occurs in most blind individuals. It can also occur in sighted individuals who live in environments with limited light exposure. This disorder has also been reported in individuals who have sustained traumatic brain injury.[8]
- Shift work disorder is reported most frequently in individuals working night shifts, early morning shifts, or rotating shifts. This is the most common circadian rhythm disorder, as up to 20% of the US population is engaged in some form of shift work.[9] For this reason, a patient's occupation should be assessed at the initial visit and will often provide clues as to the source of the patient's EDS. It should be noted that shift workers may have increased risk of cardiovascular disease and certain neoplasms.[10,11] In addition, shift workers are involved in more car accidents than non–shift workers.[12]
- Jet lag disorder results in either insomnia or EDS with symptoms of daytime impairment associated with transmeridian jet travel across at least 2 time zones. It is more common with eastward travel, as it is typically easier to delay one's circadian clock than to advance it. Jet lag is usually a self-limiting condition.

In addition to sleep diaries and actigraphy, several standardized questionnaires can be used to further characterize a patient's chronotype, or morningness-eveningness subtype.[13,14] Salivary melatonin levels can also be used.[15] PSG is not necessary to diagnose any of the circadian rhythm disorders.

Restless Leg Syndrome and Periodic Limb Movement Disorder

Restless legs syndrome (RLS), or Willis-Ekbom disease, is another condition that often presents with symptoms of insomnia and occurs in approximately 5% to 10% of the general population.[16] The 4 cardinal features of RLS include:

- An urge to move the legs often accompanied by an uncomfortable sensation
- Symptoms that worsen with rest or inactivity
- Symptoms that are relieved with movement
- Symptoms that occur predominantly in the evening hours

RLS, like circadian rhythm disorders, can present with insomnia, and many patients with this condition will not volunteer the necessary history. The sensation of lower extremity discomfort that they experience can be difficult for them to explain and has numerous descriptions in the literature. The key feature is that it is uncomfortable to the patient. One must be careful to distinguish nocturnal cramping, which is quite common in elderly patients, and neuropathic pain, which typically has a burning, tingling, or hypersensitive quality to it.

Periodic limb movements are repetitive triple flexion responses involving the great toe, ankle, and knee that occur out of sleep. These movements can sometimes lead to arousals, and if symptoms of daytime impairment are present, a diagnosis of periodic limb movement disorder (PLMD) may be considered. This diagnosis is confirmed when PSG demonstrates a periodic limb movement index of 15 or more in adults or 5 or more in children.

PLMD cannot be diagnosed in the presence of RLS or other sleep disorders such as obstructive sleep apnea (OSA) or narcolepsy. Although periodic limb movements are common in patients with RLS, if a patient describes symptoms consistent with RLS, the diagnosis of PLMD is excluded.

Sleep-Related Breathing Disorders

Loud or habitual snoring and witnessed apneas can suggest a diagnosis of OSA. In addition, patients with OSA may also describe restless sleep, frequent awakenings, nocturia, night sweats, dry mouth, or dull morning headaches. In contrast to the other disorders listed in this article, the physical examination is quite important in the evaluation of a patient with suspected OSA. This topic is discussed in more detail in the physical examination section. Patients with other sleep-related breathing disorders, such as central sleep apnea and nocturnal hypoventilation, do not always present with EDS and for the sake of brevity will not be discussed.

Narcolepsy and Other Hypersomnias of Central Origin

In contrast to patients with insomnia, RLS, or circadian rhythm disorders, a patient with a central hypersomnia has no difficulty falling asleep. Narcolepsy is the most well-described central hypersomnia, and is now subdivided into type 1 and type 2 based on cerebrospinal fluid (CSF) hypocretin (orexin)-1 levels. Type 1 patients have low or undetectable CSF hypocretin-1 levels ($\leq$110 pg/mL), whereas type 2 patients have normal CSF levels of this neuropeptide.[17] Symptoms typically develop in patients by their early 20s; however, patients presenting in their 40s have been described.[18]

In addition to EDS and sleep attacks, patients with narcolepsy may exhibit the following symptoms:

- Sleep paralysis, or the inability to move for several minutes when awakening, often accompanied by a feeling of suffocation
- Hypnagogic/hypnopompic hallucinations, which are vivid tactile, auditory, or visual hallucinations that occur either when falling asleep (hypnopompic) or when awakening (hypnagogic). Hypnagogic hallucinations are more specific to narcolepsy.
- Cataplexy, or emotionally triggered weakness of the skeletal musculature with complete preservation of consciousness. It can manifest in a variety of ways including buckling of the knees, drooping of the eyelids, and other facial muscles or, in extreme cases, total body collapse. The weakness is brief and usually resolves within several minutes. Cataplexy can be seen in both type 1 and type 2 narcolepsy, however it is more common in type 1 narcolepsy.

A key feature of the EDS in these patients is the improvement that occurs with napping. Narcoleptic patients describe naps that are refreshing, and prophylactic or planned napping is often a component of the treatment strategy. If the patient wakes up from the nap unrefreshed, an alternate diagnosis should be considered, such as idiopathic hypersomnia. Patients may also exhibit automatic behaviors, such as repetitive movements, nonsensical writing, or irrelevant speech.

Kleine-Levin syndrome is a recurrent hypersomnia associated with symptoms of hyperphagia, hypersexuality, and cognitive impairment.[19] This disorder is most prevalent in adolescents; however, it is quite rare, affecting an estimated 1 to 5 per million individuals. Patients experience symptomatic episodes lasting on average 1 to 3 weeks, with periods of intervening normal behavior. Cycles often recur every 2 to 3 months.

Menstruation-related hypersomnia is another rare episodic hypersomnia, with symptoms closely tied to the patient's the menstrual cycle.[20] Patients with menstruation-related hypersomnia do not frequently exhibit the behavioral and cognitive changes seen in patients with Kleine-Levin syndrome. If no etiology can be identified, the individual is often diagnosed with idiopathic hypersomnia. This disorder is subdivided into idiopathic hypersomnia with or without long sleep times, defined as a sleep time of 10 hours or more per night.

Parasomnias

Parasomnias are not typically associated with EDS. This includes patients with REM-behavior disorder, as well as patients with NREM parasomnias such as sleepwalking, sleep-related eating disorder, and sleep terrors.

PHYSICAL EXAMINATION

In most cases, a patient with EDS will not show specific findings on examination. Falling asleep while waiting for the physician, excessive yawning, difficulty keeping the eyes open, and poor concentration may help support the history, however, if absent does not exclude a diagnosis of EDS.

The general examination should include blood pressure, heart rate, neck circumference measurement, cardiovascular and pulmonary examination, and evaluation of the extremities for any signs of peripheral edema. Depending on the history, a more through neurologic examination may be warranted, especially if the patient presents with symptoms of a central hypersomnia disorder. Patients with OSA may have several findings to suggest a predisposition to sleep-disordered breathing. These findings are summarized in **Box 6**.

Patients with signs of peripheral neuropathy on examination should be queried for symptoms of RLS; however, it should be noted that the diagnosis of RLS is made entirely on patient history and that the examination of a patient with RLS is often normal.

ADDITIONAL TESTING

Surveys

- The Epworth Sleepiness Scale should be handed out at every patient visit. Sleep diaries may be useful in the evaluation of a patient with insomnia, insufficient sleep time, or circadian rhythm disorders.
- Chronotype questionnaires may be useful in helping characterize a patient's morningness-eveningness subtype.

Actigraphy

- Actigraphy may be useful in the evaluation of a patient with insomnia, insufficient sleep time, or circadian rhythm disorders, especially if they are unable to complete a sleep diary, for example, pediatric patients or patients with cognitive impairment.

Box 6
Physical findings seen in obstructive sleep apnea

Obesity (body mass index >30 kg/m^2)

A large neck circumference (>43.2 cm [17 in] men and >40.6 cm [16 in] women)

Turbinate hypertrophy or nasal septum deviation

Excessive oropharyngeal tissue

Tonsillar hypertrophy

Macroglossia

Tongue scalloping

High-arched palate

Retrognathia

Micrognathia

Maxillary or mandibular insufficiency

Laboratory Testing

- The DQB1*0602 haplotype is present in up to 98% of narcolepsy patients with a history of cataplexy and may be assayed from a whole blood sample. Although specific, this test lacks sensitivity, as approximately 25% of the general population also exhibits this haplotype. CSF hypocretin-1 provides a highly sensitive and specific test for the confirmation of type 1 narcolepsy, however, is not commonly used in clinical practice because of the invasive nature of the lumbar puncture.
- Serum ferritin levels should be measured in any patient with symptoms of RLS, and a value less than 50 ng/mL should be treated with iron supplementation.
- Salivary melatonin kits are now clinically available and can be used to estimate dim-light melatonin onset in a patient presenting with symptoms of a circadian rhythm disorder.
- If the patient describes symptoms consistent with fatigue, a complete blood count, electrolyte panel, thyroid function testing, and iron panel may be considered.
- A urine or serum drug screen may be indicated to rule out substance abuse.

Polysomnography, Multiple Sleep Latency Test, and Maintenance of Wakefulness Test

PSG is indicated in the evaluation of any patient with a suspected sleep-related breathing disorder, PLMD, narcolepsy, or nocturnal seizures. This test has traditionally been performed in the sleep laboratory with electrodes to monitor electroencephalographic activity, eye movements, chin electromyographic tone, chest and abdominal movement, nasal and oral airflow, snoring, oxygen saturation, heart rate, limb movements, and body position.

Home sleep testing technology has been employed recently as an alternative to traditional in-laboratory testing when sleep-disordered breathing is suspected. Several devices are available, and they differ in the number of physiologic variables measured and the algorithms used to calculate apnea-hypopnea indices. It should be noted that these devices are often less sensitive than in-laboratory PSG and are more prone to artifact and user error.

The multiple sleep latency test (MSLT) is used as a standardized measure of a patient's ability to fall asleep, and is often used to aid in the diagnosis of narcolepsy. It consists of 5 nap periods of 20 minutes each, with intervening 2-hour periods during which the patient is free to engage in nonstimulating activities.[21]

The MSLT should be preceded by an in-laboratory PSG, both to ensure at least 6 hours of nocturnal sleep time and to exclude other etiologies of EDS such sleep-disordered breathing. The MSLT typically begins 1 to 2 hours after completion of the PSG. The patient lies in a dark, quiet room and attempts to fall asleep.

Sleep-onset latency (SOL), or the time from lights out to sleep onset, is recorded for each nap period. A mean SOL of 10 minutes or less indicates sleepiness.[22] Patients with narcolepsy frequently exhibit a SOL of less than 8 minutes. If the patient enters REM sleep at any time during the nap period, it is recorded as a spontaneous onset REM period (SOREMP). The presence of at least 2 SOREMPs indicates narcolepsy. SOREMPs can also be seen in circadian rhythm disorders and sleep-related breathing disorders and in individuals with insufficient sleep time.

Medications that can affect MSLT results should be discontinued 3 to 4 weeks before testing. These medications include antidepressants, sedatives, and stimulants. Excessive caffeine use should be avoided the day before. A drug-urine screen is frequently used to exclude drugs of abuse. A 2-week sleep dairy or actigraphy is suggested to confirm the presence of a regular sleep schedule before testing. Patients should be encouraged to sleep as much as possible during the week before testing.

While the MSLT is used as a measure of an individual's ability to fall asleep, the maintenance of wakefulness test (MWT) is used as a standardized measure of an individual's ability to stay awake. It consists of 4 periods of 40 minutes each, during which the patient is placed in a dimly lit room and attempts to remain awake.[21] Like the MSLT, these periods are separated by 2-hour intervals, during which the patient is free to engage in nonstimulating

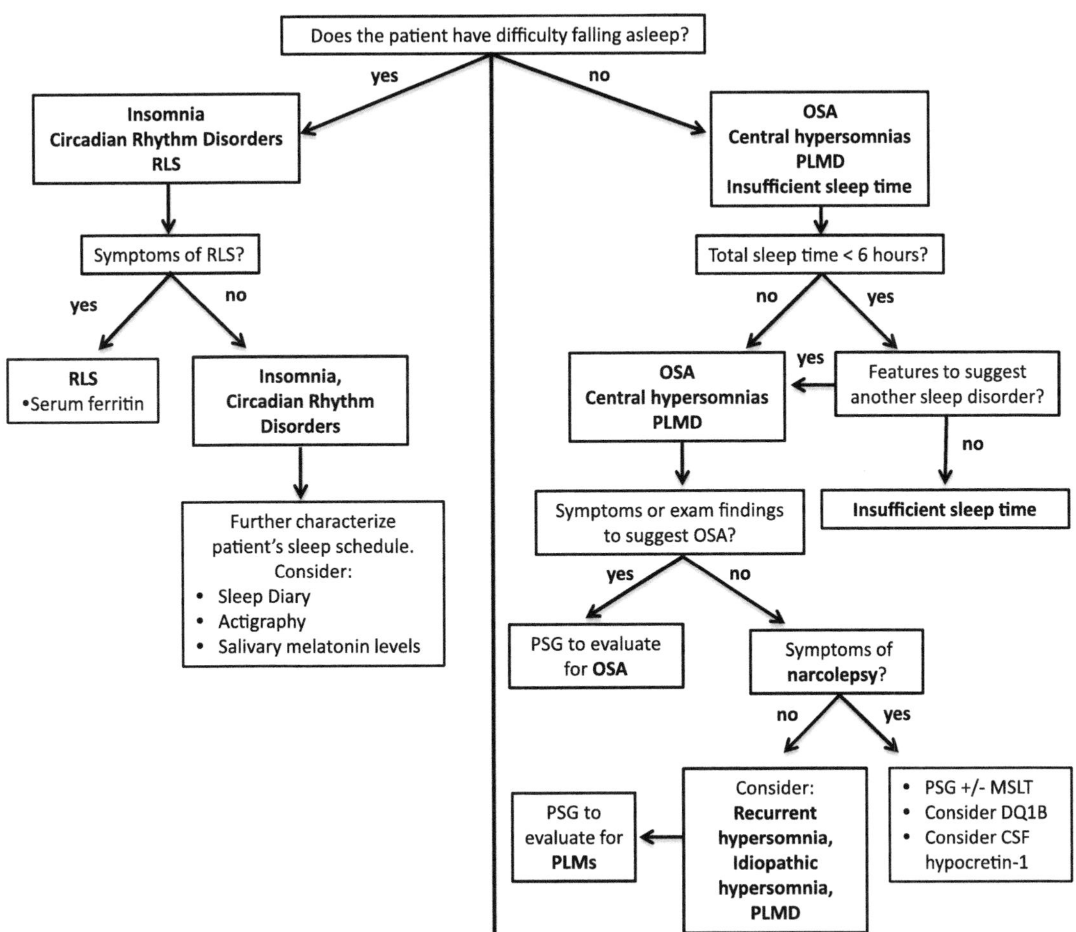

Fig. 1. Common sleep disorders to consider in any patient presenting with excessive daytime sleepiness.

activities. The test should begin no more than 3 hours after the patient's routine wake up time.

In contrast to the MSLT, a PSG is unnecessary before testing. If the patient does fall asleep, SOL is recorded. A mean SOL of less than 8 minutes usually indicates EDS.[23] In contrast to the MSLT, the MWT is not used for diagnostic purposes; however, it can be used to measure treatment response. It is most commonly used by the transportation and aviation industry to measure the alertness of commercial drivers and airline pilots.[24]

It is important to emphasize that the MSLT and MWT are not valid in isolation. They are adjunctive tests and as such should always be interpreted in light of the patient's clinical presentation. **Fig. 1** reviews common sleep disorders to consider in any patient presenting with EDS.

REFERENCES

1. Young TB. Epidemiology of daytime sleepiness: definitions, symptomatology, and prevalence. J Clin Psychiatry 2004;65(Suppl 16):12–6.
2. International classification of sleep disorders. 3rd edition. Darien (IL): American Academy of Sleep Medicine; 2014.
3. Johns MW. A new method for measuring daytime sleepiness: the Epworth Sleepiness Scale. Sleep 1991;14:540–5.
4. Rosenthal TC, Majeroni BA, Pretorius R, et al. Fatigue: an overview. Am Fam Physician 2008;78(10): 1173–9.
5. Chotinaiwattarakul W, O'Brien LM, Fan L, et al. Fatigue, tiredness, and lack of energy improve with treatment for OSA. J Clin Sleep Med 2009;5(3):222–7.
6. Ancoli-Israel S, Cole R, Alessi C, et al. The role of actigraphy in the study of sleep and circadian rhythms. Sleep 2003;26:342–92.
7. Ohayon MM. Epidemiology of insomnia: what we know and what we still need to learn. Sleep Med Rev 2002;6(2):97.
8. Ayalon L, Borodkin K, Dishon L, et al. Circadian rhythm sleep disorders following mild traumatic brain injury. Neurology 2007;68(14):1136–40.
9. Drake CL, Wright KP Jr. Shift work, shift work disorder, and jet lag. In: Kryger MH, Roth T, Dement WC, editors. Principles and practice of sleep medicine. 5th edition. Philadelphia: Elsevier Saunders; 2011. p. 784–98.
10. Boggild H, Knutsson A. Shift work, risk factors and cardiovascular disease. Scand J Work Environ Health 1999;25:85–99.
11. Knutsson A. Health disorders of shift workers. Occup Environ Med 2003;53:103–8.
12. Akerstedt T, Wright KP Jr. Sleep loss and fatigue in shift work and shift work disorder. Sleep Med Clin 2009;4(2):257–71.
13. Horne JA, Ostberg O. A self-assessment questionnaire to determine morningness-eveningness in human circadian rhythms. International Journal of Chronobiology 1976;4(2):97–110.
14. Juda M, Vetter C, Roenneberg T. The Munich chronotype questionnaire for shift-workers (MCTQShift). J Biol Rhythms 2013;28(2):130–40.
15. Voultsios A, Kennaway DJ, Dawson D. Salivary melatonin as a circadian phase marker: validation and comparison to plasma melatonin. J Biol Rhythms 1997;12(5):457–66.
16. Ohayon MM, O'Hara R, Vitiello MV. Epidemiology of restless legs syndrome: a synthesis of the literature. Sleep Med Rev 2012;16(4):283–95.
17. Mignot E, Lammers GJ, Ripley B, et al. The role of cerebrospinal fluid hypocretin measurement in the diagnosis of narcolepsy and other hypersomnias. Arch Neurol 2002;59:1553–62.
18. Leschziner G. Narcolepsy: a clinical review. Pract Neurol 2014;14(5):323–31.
19. Miglis MM, Guilleminault C. Kleine-Levin syndrome: a review. Nat Sci Sleep 2014;6:19–26.
20. Billard M, Guilleminault C, Dement WC. A menstruation-linked periodic hypersomnia: Kleine-Levin syndrome or new clinical entity. Neurology 1975;25:436–43.
21. Littner MR, Kushida C, Wise M, et al, Standards of Practice Committee of the American Academy of Sleep Medicine. Practice parameters for clinical use of the multiple sleep latency test and the maintenance of wakefulness test. Sleep 2005;28:113–21.
22. Van den Hoed J, Kraemer H, Guilleminault C, et al. Disorders of excessive daytime somnolence: polygraphic and clinical data for 100 patients. Sleep 1981;4(1):23–37.
23. Carskadon MA, Dement WC, Mitler MM, et al. Guidelines for the multiple sleep latency test (MSLT): a standard measure of sleepiness. Sleep 1986;9(4):519–24.
24. Arand D, Bonnet M, Hurwitz T, et al. The clinical use of the MSLT and MWT. Sleep 2005;28(1):123–44.

Snoring, Irregular Respiration, Hypoventilation, and Apneas

Olukayode O. Ogunrinde, MD

KEYWORDS

• Snoring • Apnea • Sleep apnea • Sleep-related breathing disorder • Obstructive sleep apnea • Central sleep apnea • Obesity hypoventilation syndrome • Irregular respiration

KEY POINTS

- Sleep-related breathing disorders (SRDBs) are common causes of sleep disturbances and impairment of daytime function.
- Snoring, apnea, irregular respiration, and hypoventilation are signs that suggest the presence of SRBDs.
- It is important that health care providers recognize and regularly ask patients about these signs, along with other symptoms that may prompt further evaluation.
- Unrecognized or untreated SRBDs can lead to significant health consequences and overall poor quality of life.
- Various diagnostic and therapeutic options are available to manage the different types of SRBDs.

INTRODUCTION

The presence of snoring, apnea, irregular respiration, and hypoventilation suggest an underlining sleep-related breathing disorder (SRBD), which if untreated can lead to significant health consequences. This article discusses how to evaluate and manage patients with signs and symptoms suggestive of SRBD.

SNORING

Snoring is a common complaint in children and adults. It is regarded as a social nuisance, but now there is mounting evidence that snoring may be associated with serious health consequences. Snoring is a sound produced by vibration of the soft tissues of the upper airway during sleep. It occurs in virtually all individuals, but habitual snoring is a health problem. Epidemiologic studies have shown that habitual snoring is common in 16% to 89% of the general population between the ages of 30 and 69 years.[1] In one study of adults 65 years and older, 30% of the men and 19% of the women reported loud snoring.[2] The male-to-female ratio is approximately 2:1. Snoring can vary in intensity and frequency nightly, and may be worse in the supine position. It can be associated with transient arousals during sleep. Snoring can occur in the absence of SRBD, especially in conditions that lead to narrowing of the upper airway, such as pregnancy, obesity, nasal congestion, hypothyroidism, acromegaly, adenotonsillar hypertrophy, and various craniofacial

Funding Sources: None.
Conflict of Interest: None.
Department of Sleep Medicine, Northwest Permanente, PC, Physician and Surgeons, Kaiser Permanente Health System, 2400 Lancaster Drive Northeast, Salem, OR 97305-1221, USA
E-mail address: Ogunox@gmail.com

Sleep Med Clin 9 (2014) 499–511
http://dx.doi.org/10.1016/j.jsmc.2014.08.002
1556-407X/14/$ – see front matter

abnormalities. Also, snoring can occur with increased weight gain.[3] Some epidemiologic studies have shown that snoring may be associated with increased risk of hypertension,[4] and cardiovascular[5] and cerebrovascular disease,[6] but the evidence is not overwhelming due to inconsistent results from other studies,[7,8] suggesting that snoring alone is not an independent risk factor. In one observational study of 110 patients, increased frequency of heavy snoring was associated with carotid artery atherosclerosis,[9] and another recent study showed similar findings.[10] Risk factors for snoring include male gender, older age, overweight, alcohol use, smoking, postmenopausal status, narrow nasal/oral cavity, broad neck, muscle relaxants, and sedative-hypnotic agents.

Clinical Evaluation

It is important to evaluate patients with habitual snoring, to determine if sleep disruption is present and to identify potential SRBD. Most patients are not aware that they snore; rather, it is noted by their bed partner. All patients should be asked about snoring, along with episodes of cessation in breathing or waking up choking or gasping for air during sleep. Other symptoms of sleep disruption include restless sleep, daytime sleepiness, fatigue, irritability, and poor concentration. The patient should be asked about mouth breathing and dryness, which suggests increased upper airway resistance. Further questioning should include use of alcohol, smoking, and medications that can contribute to increased airway narrowing or collapsibility.[11] Drugs such as muscle relaxants, barbiturates, and benzodiazepines can induce increased upper airway resistance in healthy volunteers leading to snoring.[12] Common physical examination findings include increased body mass index, larger neck circumference, narrow nasal/oral pharynx, nasal septal deviation, nasal polyps, adenotonsillar hypertrophy, swollen or hypertrophic turbinates, and other craniofacial abnormalities.

Diagnostic Evaluation

The differential diagnosis for snoring includes the following:

- Upper airway resistance syndrome (UARS)
- Obstructive sleep apnea (OSA)
- Stridor
- Sleep-related groaning (catathrenia)
- Chronic nasal congestion and other craniofacial disorders

Diagnostic testing in a patient who snores helps to confirm or exclude presence of SRBD. If OSA is suspected, polysomnograph (PSG) or portable monitor (PM) should be performed. In patients suspected of having nocturnal desaturation, overnight oximetry can be performed, and if positive, warrants further evaluation. Diagnostic evaluation for suspected craniofacial abnormalities or adenotonsillar hypertrophy may include lateral cephalometric radiographic studies or fiberoptic pharyngoscopy, which provide information about upper airway patency. If other medical conditions are suspect, laboratory or imaging studies should be performed to identify and then treat those conditions.

Treatment

It is not clear that snoring progresses to OSA. In the absence of SRBDs, treating snoring helps to minimize any sleep disturbances to patient and bed partner, and alleviate upper airway discomfort and embarrassment. Conservative treatment includes weight loss, smoking cessation, avoidance of alcohol a few hours before bedtime, and change in sleep position (nonsupine position). Weight loss should be recommended for overweight or obese patients. In one study, weight loss reduced snoring frequency and intensity.[13] Although smoking cessation is recommended, results showing correlation between snoring and smoking have been weak and inconsistent. One observational study did show increased risk of snoring among current and former smokers when compared with nonsmokers.[14] Sleeping in the lateral position can reduce snoring frequency and intensity.[15] Posture alarm devices, special pillows, and modified night wear have been used to increase the likelihood of maintaining nonsupine sleep position. Another attempt to decrease or eliminate snoring is by improving nasal patency or decreasing nasal congestion. Steroid-based intranasal spray may be helpful in snorers with chronic nasal congestion but data on long-term benefits are lacking. Furthermore, long-term benefits of lubricant nasal spray, homeopathic nasal preparations, and internal and external nasal dilators are lacking.[16]

The use of oral appliances (OAs) can reduce or eliminate snoring by increasing the size or preventing upper airway collapse during sleep. OAs, such as mandible-repositioning appliances (MRA) or tongue-retaining devices (TRDs), work by either advancing the mandible or protruding the tongue to enlarge the oropharyngeal cavity. OAs are highly effective if used properly and fabricated by a dentist with expertise in treating sleep apnea.[17] Common side effects include teeth discomfort, teeth movement, bite changes, temporomandibular joint (TMJ) pain, xerostomia, and excessive salivation. Dental follow-up is recommended to assess for these potential problems and to manage appropriately. The use of positive airway pressure (PAP) therapy (eg, continuous PAP [CPAP]) is an effective and a safe treatment for snoring. Unfortunately, the Centers for Medicare and Medicaid Services (CMS) and all private health insurers do not cover the cost of PAP therapy for treatment of snoring.

For patients who have failed conservative methods, or cannot tolerate OA or PAP therapy, surgery is another alternative option. Surgical intervention involves removal or modification of soft tissue in the nasal oral cavity. Nasal turbinate reduction, nasal valve surgery, and septoplasty are procedures that help decrease resistance in the nasal passage. For surgical intervention to the oropharyngeal cavity, uvulopalatopharyngoplasty (UPPP) has been performed in many patients. It involves surgical removal of soft palate, uvula, tonsillar pillars, and tonsils if present. In one study, snoring was significantly reduced or eliminated in 60 (87%) of 69 patients after UPPP, but after 13 months, the success rate dropped to 46%.[18] In another study, no significant change in snoring frequency or intensity was found, but some patients and their bed partner did report subjective improvements in sleep quality.[19] UPPP does cause some discomfort in the immediate period after surgery, and potential complications include nasal reflux, painful pharyngeal wall scarring, dysphonia, infection, and bleeding. Uvulopalatal flap, laser-assisted uvulopalatopharyngoplasty (LAUP), and radiofrequency palate surgery are all modified versions of the UPPP procedure, to help mitigate complication. Convincing evidence supporting long-term benefit of any surgical intervention for snoring is lacking. Despite mounting evidence that snoring may be associated with carotid artery atherosclerosis, and limited data showing increased risk of cardiovascular disease, treatment for snoring alone is not covered by any health care insurance agency.

APNEA

Sleep apnea (SA) can occur in both children and adults, and the incidence increases with older age. The increase in obesity, with 35.7% of adults being obese,[20] has led to an increase in the prevalence of SA. The estimated incidence of SA in the US adult population is approximately 16%.[21] A growing body of evidence indicates that SA is associated with increased risk of the following:

- Coronary artery disease[22]
- Congestive heart failure (CHF)[22]
- Cardiac dysrhythmias[23]
- Hypertension[24]
- Stroke[25]
- Diabetes[26]
- Metabolic syndrome[27]
- Depression[28]
- Cognitive impairment[29]
- Motor vehicle crash[30]
- Perioperative complications[31]
- Death[32]

According to the international classification of sleep disorders, apnea during sleep can be categorized as

- Obstructive apnea
- Central apnea
- Mixed apnea
- Hypopnea
- Respiratory effort related arousal (RERA)[33]

The description is based on their morphology on PSG.[34] Apnea is the cessation or near cessation of airflow lasting at least 10 seconds in duration. It is OA if ventilatory effort persists during an event, and it is central apnea if ventilatory effort is absent. Mixed apnea means that there is an interval during which respiratory effort is absent, and then partially restored at the end of an event. Hypopnea is reduction in airflow to a degree that does not meet the criteria of an apnea. The definition of hypopnea has changed over time and the currently accepted definition is airflow reduction of at least 30% from pre-event baseline, lasting at least 10 seconds, associated with at least 3% to 4% desaturation and/or an arousal. The American Academy Of Sleep Medicine (AASM) recognizes the 3% to 4% desaturation rule, but CMS recognizes only the 4% rule.[34] RERAs are defined as a sequence of breaths lasting 10 seconds, associated with increasing respiratory effort or flattening of the nasal pressure waveform, terminated by an arousal from sleep, and does not meet criteria for an apnea or hypopnea. The frequency of apnea, hypopnea, and RERAs is reported as apnea-hypopnea index (AHI) or respiratory disturbance index (RDI). UARS is a subtype of OSA and is defined mainly by RERAs in a symptomatic patient. Complex sleep apnea is a variant of central sleep apnea (CSA), characterized by the emergence or persistence of central apnea during PAP titration for treatment of OSA. It tends to occur in 10% to 20% of patients and usually spontaneously resolves within 8 to 12 weeks in most patients.[35] A complete list of terms and definitions can be seen in **Box 1**.

Box 1
Clinical definition of sleep-related breathing disorders

Apnea (A): >90% cessation of airflow for >10 seconds

Hypopnea (H): >30% cessation of airflow for >10 seconds with 3%–4% decrease in oxygen saturation and/or arousal

Apnea-hypopnea index (AHI): Total of apnea and hypopnea events recorded per hour of sleep or recording time

Respiratory disturbance index (RDI): Total of apnea, hypopnea, and respiratory effort related arousal (RERA) events per hour of sleep or recording time

Mild obstructive sleep apnea (OSA): ≥ AHI or RDI 5–15/h

Moderate OSA: AHI or RDI ≥15–30/h

Severe OSA: AHI or RDI ≥30 h

Obstructive sleep apnea syndrome (OSAS): AHI or RDI ≥15/h or ≥5/h with symptoms of disrupted sleep

Central sleep apnea syndrome (CSAS): AHI ≥5 with symptoms of disrupted sleep

Upper airway resistance syndrome (UARS): presence of RERAs with symptoms of disrupted sleep

Complex sleep apnea syndrome: Emergence or persistence of central respiratory events during positive airway pressure titration for treatment of OSA

Obesity hypoventilation syndrome: $Paco_2$ greater than 45 mm Hg, Pao_2 less than 70 mm Hg, body mass index (BMI) ≥30 kg/m^2 with sleep apnea and lack of other cause of hypercapnia

Obstructive Sleep Apnea

OSA is the most common of all SRBDs. It is characterized by partial or complete collapse of the upper airway, causing fluctuation in oxygen saturation and sleep fragmentation. The proposed mechanism appears to be impaired neuronal input that serves to resist airway collapses or withdrawal of neuronal input to pharyngeal dilator muscles.[36] In the United States, the prevalence of OSA is estimated to be 3% to 7% in men and 2% to 5% in women,[37] and more than 80% of adults are yet to be diagnosed.[38] It is more common in men than women but the incidence is approximately the same in both men and postmenopausal women. The major risk factors for OSA include obesity, being male, and older age. The strongest risk factor regardless of age is obesity. In one large prospective study of 690 patients, a 10% increase in weight gain was associated with a sixfold increase in the odds of developing OSA.[39] Few studies have shown increase in OSA in African American when compared with white individuals of the same age, independent of weight.[40] Also, there is increased prevalence of OSA among Asians, mostly attributed to craniofacial anatomy.[41] A complete list of risk factors for OSA is listed in **Box 2**.

Central Sleep Apnea

Central apnea can be a benign finding in healthy individuals (especially in children), and tends to occur during transition from wakefulness to sleep or after an arousal during sleep.[42] CSA is a disorder characterized by repetitive cessation of both airflow and ventilatory effort during sleep. CSA is estimated to be approximately 10% of all sleep apnea cases. In the general population, the prevalence of CSA is less than 1% and incidence is higher among the elderly.[43] Risk factors for CSA include male gender, CHF, stroke, neurodegenerative disease, and chronic opioid medication use. CSA can be primary (idiopathic) or secondary (ie, CHF, stroke, high altitude, or drugs). The underlying pathophysiology of CSA is related to either hyperventilation or hypoventilation.[44] In patients with CHF, opiate drug use, or high altitude sickness, central apnea is due to posthypocapnia hyperventilation. Respiration during sleep is mostly driven by partial pressure of arterial carbon dioxide ($Paco_2$). Hyperventilation leads to a drop in $Paco_2$ levels below the apneic threshold, a level below which respiration ceases. Breathing resumes again

Box 2
Risk factors for sleep-related breathing disorders

- Older age
- Increased BMI (>30 kg/m^2, large waist circumference)
- Gender (men > women)
- Menopausal women
- Snoring
- Larger neck girth (>17 inches for men, >16 inches for women)
- Ethnicity (African American > White)
- Family history of OSA
- Small and/or abnormality craniofacial structural
- Use of alcohol/sedatives
- Smoking

when $Paco_2$ level rises above the apneic threshold. Central apnea due to hypoventilation occurs when there is impairment of wakefulness stimulus to breathe during sleep and/or impaired neuromuscular ventilatory response. This can be seen in patients with central nervous system disease, neuromuscular disease, or chest wall disorders. CSA can coexist with OSA in certain patients.

Clinical Evaluation

Clinical symptoms and signs of SA can be elicited during a clinic visit or routine health maintenance evaluation. A comprehensive sleep evaluation should include detailed sleep history, sleep questionnaires, physical examination, and diagnostic testing.[45] In patients suspected of having SA, the most common symptom is daytime sleepiness. Further careful questioning should include timing and pattern of feeling sleepy (ie, falling asleep in boring, passive, or monotonous situations). Also, the patient should be asked about snoring, witnessed apnea, and waking up gasping or choking for air during sleep. Other signs and symptoms suggestive of SA are outlined in **Box 3**. Questions about sleep disturbance should be asked in high-risk populations (ie, commercial drivers). Commercial drivers should be asked about recent motor vehicle crashes or near-misses due to falling asleep. Other patient populations that have increase risk of SA are listed in **Box 4**. On physical examination, patients with SA usually have a large body habitus (BMI >30 kg/m2) with increased waist girth, large neck, and a crowded nasal/oral pharynx. Detailed physical examination findings are listed in **Box 5**.

Several screening questionnaires have been developed to try to identify patients at high risk for SA. These questionnaires have been validated only to screen patients with OSA. Details of each questionnaire are not discussed in this article.

Box 3
Sign and symptoms of sleep-related breathing disorders

- Snoring
- Witnessed apnea
- Choking or gasping for air
- Fatigue
- Restless or fragmented sleep
- Daytime sleepiness or somnolence
- Morning headache
- Moodiness or irritability
- Impaired concentration or inattention
- Memory disturbance
- Drowsy driving
- Dry mouth or sore throat
- Nocturia
- Nocturnal dyspnea
- Nocturnal panic attacks
- Nocturnal angina
- Palpitation
- Myalgia
- Decrease libido/erectile dysfunction
- Bruxism
- Insomnia

Box 4
High-risk populations that should evaluated for sleep-related breathing disorders

- Patients with any of the following conditions:
  - Coronary artery disease
  - Congestive heart failure
  - Cor pulmonale
  - Cardiac dysrhythmias (eg, atrial fibrillation)
  - Refractory hypertension
  - Stroke
  - Diabetes
  - Metabolic syndrome
  - Psychiatric disorders (eg, depression)
  - End-stage renal disease
  - Hypotestosteronism
  - Hypothyroidism
  - Acromegaly
  - Down syndrome
  - Glaucoma
  - Polycythemia
  - Polycystic ovarian syndrome
  - Neurologic disorders (Parkinson, multiple system atrophy, amyotrophic lateral sclerosis, epilepsy)
  - Chronic lung disease (eg, pulmonary hypertension, chronic obstructive pulmonary disease, asthma)
  - Preoperative for bariatric and other major surgeries requiring general anesthesia
- Pregnant women
- Commercial drivers (pilots, bus or truck drivers)

Box 5
Physical examination findings in patients with sleep-related breathing disorders

- Obesity (BMI >30 kg/m^2)
- Neck girth (>17 for men, >16 for women)
- Retrognathia
- Micrognathia
- Macroglossia
- Hypertrophic tonsils/adenoids
- Extended or redundant soft palate
- Enlarged or elongated uvula
- High arched or narrow hard palate
- Enlarged nasal turbinate
- Deviated nasal septum
- Wide nasal alar
- Elevated morning blood pressure

Because sleepiness is the most common presenting symptom of OSA, the Epworth sleepiness scale (ESS) is the most used and readily available.[46] Other questionnaires, such as Berlin, STOP-BANG, and American Society of Anesthesiologists are frequently used and have proven to be very effective in identifying high-risk patients.[47]

Diagnostic Evaluation

A variety of conditions can cause sleep disturbance, mimicking symptoms that are found in patients with SA. The differential diagnosis for SA includes the following:

- Primary snoring
- UARS
- Chronic lung disease
- Hypoventilation syndromes
- Narcolepsy
- Gastroesophageal reflux disease
- Hypothyroidism
- Periodic limb movement disorder
- Insomnia
- Neuromuscular disease
- Neurodegenerative disease
- Chronic opiate therapy
- High-altitude periodic breathing

SA often presents with an array of neurocognitive, behavioral, and cardiovascular consequences that warrant further evaluation. Clinical evaluation and screening questionnaires are not enough to establish or exclude a particular diagnosis. Diagnostic tests should be performed only after a comprehensive sleep evaluation. The high-risk patient population (see **Box 4**) with symptoms of sleep disturbance and/or patients not responding to therapies for their primary health condition should be screened for SA. Because of the high prevalence of SA in the surgical population, screening should be performed in those patients.[31] Before testing, all patients should be educated about the pathophysiology, risk factors, and clinical consequences of SA. PSG and PM are currently the only approved testing for SA. PSG is the gold standard for evaluating patients with sleep disorders but may not always be readily available. PSG should be done in a standardized AASM-accredited sleep laboratory with video multichannel recordings that determine sleep time, sleep stages, body position, snoring, airflow, heart rate, oxygen saturation, and limb movements. PM is approved for use in an unattended setting. The PSG or PM test should be performed under the supervision of board-certified sleep specialists or clinicians trained in sleep medicine.[48] The use of PM may underestimate the severity of events when compared with PSG because calculation of RDI or AHI is based on total recording time rather than total sleep time. PM should be done only in patients with a high pretest probability of moderate to severe OSA, and should not be used in patients with significant comorbid conditions (ie, significant cardiopulmonary diseases) or if other sleep disorders are suspected.[48] There are multiple approved devices on the market, but all PM devices should have at least airflow, respiratory effort, and oximetry sensors. PSG should be performed in a symptomatic patient with a negative PM study. PM can be used to monitor response to non-CPAP therapies (ie, oral appliance, surgery, weight loss). If PSG or PM is performed, it should be interpreted by a board-certified sleep specialist. Routine laboratory testing is not helpful in confirming or excluding the diagnosis of SA but can be helpful in evaluating for conditions that increase risk for SA (eg, hypothyroidism).

Treatment

Treatment for SA is lifelong and usually requires a medical, surgical, or behavioral approach. Treatment should be based on patient's preference, severity of SA, potential side effects, and efficacy of therapy. The goal of treatment should be to resolve all SA-related symptoms and decrease risk of health-related consequences.

Positive airway pressure

PAP is the most effective therapy, and treatment of choice for SA. It is used as a stent to keep the upper airway open. The effect of PAP therapy in reduction of AHI and decreasing morbidity and mortality has been well documented.[49] It can be delivered in continuous (CPAP), bi-level (BPAP), or auto-titrating (APAP) mode. It is preferred that PAP therapy should be initiated after an attended full-night or split-night (diagnostic–titration) PSG.[45] APAP is approved for use in an unattended situation. It is not recommended for use without a formal titration study in patients with significant comorbid conditions (eg, CHF, chronic obstructive pulmonary disease, CSA, or hypoventilation).[50] Almost all treatment is started with CPAP. BPAP can be used in patients who have not responded well to or are intolerant of CPAP.[50] For patients with CSA, CPAP is also indicated as the initial therapy. If the patient does not respond appropriately, BPAP ST (BPAP with a backup rate) or adaptive servo-ventilation (ASV) should be introduced.[51] ASV is a modified PAP delivery system. All the devices come with pressure-relief features and humidifier to enhance comfort. PAP is delivered by a mask through a nasal, oral, or oronasal interface. The masks come in different designs and sizes to optimize comfort. Successful treatment is based on adequate compliance. Compliance is defined as any PAP device used for at least 4 hours per night, for at least 70% of the night, and at least 30 days consecutively. Education about the benefits of PAP therapy and potential problems, along with close monitoring, especially in the first few weeks of treatment is vital to adequate use and benefit.[45] Once the patient is stable on PAP therapy, yearly follow-up with a sleep physician or trained clinician is recommended. Patients undergoing surgical procedures should continue PAP therapy the night before surgery and postoperatively until full recovery from anesthesia and alertness is achieved.

Oral appliance

Another treatment option for OSA is an OA. OAs include the use of MRA or TRD. MRA is more preferred than TRD. Although not as efficacious, OA is sometimes preferred over PAP therapy. It well tolerated in most patients and efficacy varies among studies due to type of device used, OSA severity, positionality of OSA severity, degree of protrusion, and severity of BMI.[52] Treatment success is defined as AHI less than 5 or 50% reduction in AHI from baseline. Success rate with OA varies from 42% to 65%, depending on the study.[52] Efficacy is better in nonobese patients with mild to moderate OSA. Indications for OA therapy include preference for OAs over PAP, poor respond or contraindication to PAP, or failure of behavioral measures (ie, weight loss, positional therapy).[45] Before treatment with OA, a comprehensive dental evaluation is required. Potential candidates must have adequate healthy teeth and jaw mobility. Some contraindications to treatment with OA include periodontal disease, TMJ discomfort, wearing of dentures, or significant gag reflex. OA should be fitted only by qualified dental personnel with training or experience in patients with OSA. All patients fitted with OAs should be assessed for comfort, adequate device titration, and adherence. It is recommended that once the OA titration goal is achieved, PSG or PM should be performed to assess efficacy.[45] A recent meta-analysis did show that OA may have some modest effect on blood pressure lowering.[53] OA is not approved for treatment in patients with CSA. Another emerging alternative therapy for OSA is nasal expiratory positive airway pressure (EPAP), which is a device placed on the nostrils to increase resistance on expiration, thereby creating a positive pressure that prevents upper airway collapse. A few studies show that it is effective in reducing OSA severity, and it improves subjective daytime sleepiness.[54]

Surgical procedures

Surgical procedures may be considered as a secondary treatment for OSA if PAP or OA is intolerable or contraindicated. Surgical therapies include a variety of upper airway surgeries, such as UPPP (including variant uvulopalatal flap and LAUP), septoplasty, rhinoplasty, nasal valve surgery, nasal turbinate reduction surgery, palatal implants, tongue reduction surgery, genioglossus advancement, hyoid suspension, and maxillomandibular advancement surgery (MMA). A meta-analysis showed that MMA is the most effective of all surgical procedures, with a success rate defined as AHI less than 20 and/or reduction in AHI by greater than 50%.[55] The diagnosis and severity of OSA must be established, followed by a comprehensive evaluation before surgery. The patient's medical, psychological, or social well-being must be assessed, and surgical options, success rate, goals of treatment, side effects, and complications must be discussed. Surgery or OA is not effective in treatment of patients with CSA. When a patient cannot tolerate any approved therapy, and if OSA is life-threatening, tracheostomy should be considered. Although rarely performed these days, tracheostomy is effective for treatment of OSA.[56]

Behavioral therapy

Behavioral therapy for OSA includes the following:

- Weight loss
- Positional therapy (avoiding supine position)
- Avoidance of alcohol/medications that increase airway collapsibility

Weight loss should be recommended in all obese patients with SA. In one study, weight loss was effective in decreasing sleep apnea burden, especially in patients with mild OSA.[57] A PSG or PM should be performed in patients who have had significant weight loss (>10% or more of body weight) to assess severity of residual OSA and/or make adjustment to PAP therapy.

Positional therapy should be recommended for patients in whom most respiratory events occur while sleeping supine. There are many devices on the market (eg, special pillows, back pack, specialized T shirts with back pocket) that have been developed to help maintain a nonsupine sleeping position.

Adjunctive therapies

Adjunctive therapies include bariatric surgery, pharmacologic agents, and oxygen therapy. In patients with OSA who are obese, bariatric surgery should be considered as an adjunct therapy to achieve significant weight reduction and to decrease OSA burden. A meta-analysis assessing the effects of surgical weight loss on OSA showed that bariatric surgery significantly reduces AHI severity, but some patients may still have residual disease. Patients should be advised that surgical weight loss intervention may not lead to cure.[58] Oxygen therapy is not recommended as primary treatment for OSA, but can be used as an adjunct therapy if indicated. There is evidence to support nocturnal oxygen therapy for the treatment of CSA related to CHF.[51] A recent meta-analysis showed that supplemental oxygen therapy does improve oxygen saturation in patients with OSA, but the same study found that the use of oxygen only may prolong duration of apnea/hypopnea and may worsen nocturnal hypercapnia in patients with comorbid chronic respiratory disease.[59] There is no strong evidence to support the use of pharmacotherapy for treatment of OSA or CSA. Some studies have suggested that acetazolamide, theophylline, zolpidem, and triazolam may benefit certain patients with CSA.[51] For patients with residual daytime sleepiness despite effective PAP therapy, modafinil or armodafinil is effective and has been approved for use to help maintain daytime alertness.[60,61] The patient should be evaluated for other potential causes of sleepiness before initiation of these medications.

IRREGULAR RESPIRATION

Disruption of central respiratory command centers can lead to an irregular respiration pattern, which becomes more pronounced during sleep. Irregular respiration can be observed during sleep in patients with SRBD, but most often it is associated with other underlying medical conditions (eg, brainstem lesions, cardiopulmonary disorder, metabolic derailment, chronic opiate therapy).

Some of the more recognized irregular respiratory patterns are periodic breathing, ataxic breathing, apneustic breathing, and Cheyne-Stokes respiration (CSR). Periodic breathing is characterized by regular cyclic changes in tidal volumes without a period of apnea.[62] This type of breathing can occur in infants (attributed to immaturity of brain respiratory centers) and also in adults with cardiopulmonary disorders. Ataxic breathing is a rare respiratory pattern characterized by complete irregularity of breathing rate and depth, with irregular pauses.[62] It usually occurs in patients with medullar stroke or neurodegenerative disorder. Apneustic breathing is characterized by prolonged deep inspiration that ends in a pause, followed by brief expiratory phase.[62] This pattern of breathing is seen in patients with pontine stroke or mass. CSR is the most common of all, and is often associated with CSA. The rest of the discussion on irregular respiration will focus on CSR.

CSR has been well described in patients with CHF, with prevalence estimated to be approximately 30% to 40% of the adult population.[63,64] It can occur in patients with stroke, traumatic brain injury, brain tumor, opiate medication use, or metabolic derailment (eg, chronic renal disease). CSR is defined as episodes of consecutive central apneas and/or hypopneas separated by a crescendo and decrescendo pattern change in breathing amplitude, usually lasting a cycle length of 40 seconds or longer. Risk factors for CSR are male gender, older age, heart failure, and hypocapnic conditions. In patients with CHF, the pathogenesis of CSR is felt to be due to the posthypocapnia hyperventilation mechanism that was described earlier. CSR-CSA is associated with increased risk of nocturnal arrhythmias, and is associated with higher mortality rate in patients with CHF.[65]

Clinical Evaluation

Detailed sleep history should be obtained from the patient and bed partner. The bed partner may notice irregular breathing pattern during sleep. The patient should be asked about symptoms of disrupted sleep (listed in **Box 3**). Patients with underlying cardiopulmonary disease may report palpitation, paroxysmal nocturnal dyspnea, angina, or panic attacks. There are no specific physical examination signs for patients with irregular respiration. Cardiopulmonary examination may reveal irregular heart rhythm, peripheral edema, and jugular venous distension. If irregular respiration is due to an intracranial process, disturbance of cognitive function or sensory, motor, or other focal neurologic deficit may be found on examination.

Diagnostic Evaluation

The differential diagnosis for a patient with irregular respiration includes the following:

- OSA
- CSA
- Stroke
- Brain lesions
- Neurodegenerative disorders
- Neuromuscular disorders
- Cardiopulmonary disorders
- Drug or substance intoxication
- Metabolic derailment

If the exact cause of irregular respiration is known, then diagnostic testing should be directed at evaluating for comorbid SRDB. PSG should be performed and it also helps to characterize breathing pattern. If a split-night PSG is performed, the appropriate treatment modality to support ventilation can be implemented. The use of PM is not appropriate in this patient population. If underlying cardiopulmonary disorder is suspected, arterial blood gas (ABG) may shows gaseous exchange abnormality. Other diagnostic tests if indicated should include brain-imaging studies, chest radiographs, echocardiogram, electrocardiogram, and pulmonary function test.

Treatment

Treatment for irregular respiration should be tailored to each patient depending on the underlying condition. Optimization of therapy for the underlying conditions help to control, and may resolve the irregular respiration. Because CSR-CSA is common in patients with CHF, treatment of heart failure with medical therapy, cardiac transplantation, or cardiac resynchronization therapy (ie, biventricular pacing) is essential. Treatment directed at CSR-CSA, includes use of CPAP, BPAP ST, ASV, nocturnal oxygen therapy, and medications. In one prospective, randomized controlled study, the use of CPAP for the treatment of CSR-CSA in patients with CHF showed an overall reduction in AHI, improved left ventricular ejection fraction, and increased nocturnal oxygen saturation and physical endurance. However, CPAP had no effect on transplant-free survival.[66] If there is no adequate response to CPAP, then BPAP ST or ASV should be implemented. There is growing evidence that suggests ASV may be superior to all other therapies for treatment of CSR-CSA. Studies have shown that ASV reduces AHI severity, improves cardiac function and exercise endurance, and may decrease risk of future cardiac events.[66,67] Few studies have shown that nocturnal oxygen supplementation reduces AHI and improves left ventricular function in patients with CSR.[51] There is limited convincing evidence available to support the routine use of medications, such as theophylline and acetazolamide, in patients with periodic breathing or CSR.[51]

HYPOVENTILATION

Hypoventilation is characterized as $Paco_2$ retention higher than normal value. Hypoventilation can be more pronounced during sleep as respiratory drive decreases. According to the recent AASM scoring manual, hypoventilation is defined as increase in $Paco_2$ level greater than 55 mm Hg for 10 minutes or more or 10-mm Hg increase in $Paco_2$ during sleep compared with awake supine, to a value exceeding 50 mm Hg for 10 minutes or longer.[34]

Hypoventilation is seen in several conditions, such as neuromuscular disease, chronic pulmonary disease, obesity hypoventilation syndrome (OHS), congenital central hypoventilation syndrome, restrictive thoracic cage disorders (RTCD), and chronic opiate therapy. Of all these disorders, the most commonly seen in sleep clinics is OHS (formally called Pickwickian syndrome). OHS is characterized by daytime $Paco_2$ greater than 45 mm Hg and $Paco_2$ less than 70 mm Hg, in patients with BMI of 30 kg/m^2 or higher and without other cause of hypercapnia.[68] More than 90% of patients with OHS have OSA and the prevalence of OHS is estimated to be 10% to 20% among adults. Men and women are equally affected, and some studies suggest that prevalence may be higher in African American individuals because of their increased obesity rate.[69] Several proposed factors contribute to the pathogenesis of OHS, including increased airway collapsibility due to OSA, increased work of breathing, reduction in respiratory muscle strength and endurance, blunted central respiratory response, and insensitivity of neurohumoral modulator (leptin), which may contribute to $Paco_2$ elevation.[69] Hypoventilation tends to be worse during rapid eye movement (REM) sleep than non-REM sleep because of further loss of muscle tone.

Clinical Evaluation

The presenting signs and symptoms of patients with OHS are similar to those of a patient with SA. The complaint of somnolence is almost universal in patients with OHS, and they tend to have higher ESS scores. Other presenting symptoms are listed in **Box 3**. It is not uncommon for patients with OHS to complain of dyspnea on exertion and fatigability, which may be early signs of cardiopulmonary dysfunction. Physical examination findings are similar to patients with OSA (see **Box 5**). Suspicion for OHS should be high if the patient is obese and has unexplained low oxygen saturation on room air. Some patients also may present with lower extremity edema or jugular venous distension, suggestive of cor pulmonale.

Diagnostic Evaluation

Differential diagnosis for hypoventilation syndrome includes OSA, CSA, RTCD, neurodegenerative disorders, neuromuscular disorder, cardiopulmonary disorder, chronic opiate therapy, drug or substance intoxication, diaphragmatic paralysis, hypothyroidism, and metabolic derailment (eg, chronic renal failure). If suspicion for OHS is high, performing a routine ABG should show hypercapnia, hypoxemia, and a normal alveolar-arterial oxygen gradient. In few cases, complete blood count may show polycythemia, indicating a reaction to chronic hypoxemia. Elevated serum bicarbonate may indicate chronic hypercapnia. Patients with OHS should undergo PSG, which usually shows oxygen saturation below 90% during the entire sleep duration. Transcutaneous or end-tidal CO2 monitoring can be used during PSG to monitor $Paco_2$. Other diagnostic studies that should be performed to exclude or evaluate for comorbid conditions include thyroid-stimulating test, chest radiograph, pulmonary function test, electrocardiograph, and echocardiograph.

Treatment

OHS has a negative impact on quality of life, with increased morbidity and mortality rates.[69] Patients with OHS are more likely to be hospitalized for developing conditions such as acute respiratory failure, angina pectoris, pneumonia, CHF, cor pulmonale, and pulmonary hypertension.[70] Early diagnosis of OHS is very important, and treatment should be initiated without delay to avoid adverse outcome.

An in-laboratory titration study is recommended before initiation of PAP therapy. CPAP is the initial treatment option and is very effective in patients with uncomplicated OHS.[71] Patients with persistent hypoxemia may respond better to BPAP. BPAP should be initiated if the patient is intolerant to high pressures of CPAP (>15 cm H_2O) and/or if hypoxemia persists.[72] There is evidence that certain patients may respond better with use of average volume assured pressure support ventilation (AVAPS), a device that delivers a more consistent tidal volume and minute ventilation over fixed pressure support.[73] One randomized controlled study showed that the effects of AVAPS are similar to BPAP.[74] Hypercapnia usually starts to resolve within in 2 to 4 weeks. Serum bicarbonate level can be used to monitor response to treatment if the patient is not on thiazide or loop diuretics, which can falsely elevate levels. Some patients may still require nocturnal oxygen use after initiation of PAP therapy. Supplemental oxygen is recommended in patients with SpO2 less than 88% for longer than 5 minutes, despite adequate PAP use.[72] It is important to make sure that patients are compliant with PAP therapy, because oxygen may not be required over time.

Bariatric surgery should be considered in patients with OHS and morbid obesity. In one study of patients with OHS who underwent bariatric surgery, reduction in $Paco_2$ level was observed with weight loss, but $Paco_2$ level increased after 5 years at follow-up because of weight gain and worsening of OSA.[75] In patients who cannot tolerate PAP therapy and have significant disease burden, tracheostomy with ventilatory support should be considered. The use of respiratory stimulant agents has been suggested as an adjunct therapy in patients with OHS. There is very limited evidence to support routine use of respiratory stimulant agents such as medroxyprogesterone[76] and acetazolamide.[77] Medroxyprogesterone stimulates respiration through the effect on the hypothalamus, whereas acetazolamide increases minute ventilation by inducing metabolic acidosis through carbonic anhydrase inhibition. Potential side effects of these medications and the lack of overwhelming evidence have limited their use. Patients with OHS should be advised to abstain from alcohol and tobacco use. Benzodiazepine, opiates, and barbiturate medications should be avoided or used with caution.

SUMMARY

The prevalence of SRDBs is increasing, partly because of an aging population and obesity epidemic. The presence of snoring, apnea, irregular respiration, and hypoventilation suggest underlining SRBD. SRDBs are a common cause of sleep disturbances and daytime impairment. It is important that health care providers recognize these signs because if unrecognized or untreated, SRDB can lead to significant health consequences and overall poor quality of life. PSG is the preferred diagnostic testing for evaluating patients with SRBD. There are various effective treatment options available involving a medical, behavioral, or surgical approach.

REFERENCES

1. Stoohs RA, Blum HC, Haselhorst M, et al. Normative data on snoring. Eur Respir J 1998;11(2):451–7.
2. Enright PL, Newman AB, Wahl PW, et al. Prevalence and correlates of snoring and observed apneas in 5,201 older adults. Sleep 1996;19(7):531–8.
3. Berger G, Berger R, Oksenberg A. Progression of snoring and obstructive sleep apnoea: the role of increasing weight and time. Eur Respir J 2009;33:338–45.
4. Gislason T, Benediktsdóttir B, Björnsson JK, et al. Snoring, hypertension, and the sleep apnea syndrome. An epidemiologic survey of middle-aged women. Chest 1993;103:1147–51.
5. Endeshaw Y, Rice TB, Schwartz AV, et al. Snoring, daytime sleepiness, and incident cardiovascular disease in the health, aging, and body composition study. Sleep 2013;36(11):1737–45.
6. Spriggs DA, French JM, Murdy JM, et al. Snoring increases the risk of stroke and adversely affects prognosis. Q J Med 1992;83(303):555–62.
7. Yeboah J, Redline S, Johnson C, et al. Association between sleep apnea, snoring, incident cardiovascular events and all-cause mortality in an adult population: MESA. Atherosclerosis 2011;219(2):963–8.
8. Marshall NS, Wong KK, Cullen SR, et al. Snoring is not associated with all-cause mortality, incident cardiovascular disease, or stroke in the Busselton Health Study. Sleep 2012;35(9):1235–40.
9. Lee SA, Amis TC, Byth K, et al. Heavy snoring as a cause of carotid artery atherosclerosis. Sleep 2008;31:1207–13.
10. Li Y, Liu J, Wang W, et al. Association of self-reported snoring with carotid artery intima-media thickness and plaque. J Sleep Res 2012;21:87–93.
11. Riemann R, Volk R, Müller A, et al. The influence of nocturnal alcohol ingestion on snoring. Eur Arch Otorhinolaryngol 2010;267(7):1147–56.
12. Masuda A, Haji A, Wakasugi M, et al. Differences in midazolam-induced breathing patterns in healthy volunteers. Acta Anaesthesiol Scand 1995;39:785–90.
13. Braver HM, Block AJ, Perri MG. Treatment for snoring. Combined weight loss, sleeping on side, and nasal spray. Chest 1995;107:1283–8.
14. Franklin KA, Gíslason T, Omenaas E, et al. The influence of active and passive smoking on habitual snoring. Am J Respir Crit Care Med 2004;170:799–803.
15. Nakano H, Ikeda T, Hayashi M, et al. Effects of body position on snoring in apneic and nonapneic snorers. Sleep 2003;26:169–72.
16. Meoli AL, Rosen CL, Kristo D, et al. Nonprescription treatments of snoring or obstructive sleep apnea: an evaluation of products with limited scientific evidence. Sleep 2003;26:619–24.
17. Kushida CA, Morgenthaler TI, Littner MR, et al. Practice parameters for the treatment of snoring and obstructive sleep apnea with oral appliances: an update for 2005. Sleep 2006;29(2):240–3.
18. Levin BC, Becker GD. Uvulopalatopharyngoplasty for snoring: long-term results. Laryngoscope 1994;104(9):1150–2.
19. Miljeteig H, Mateika S, Haight JS, et al. Subjective and objective assessment of uvulopalatopharyngoplasty for treatment of snoring and obstructive sleep apnea. Am J Respir Crit Care Med 1994;150:1286–90.
20. Ogden CL, Carroll MD, Kit BK, et al. Prevalence of obesity in the United States (2009–2010). Hyattsville, MD: NCHS data brief, no 82. National Center for Health Statistics; 2012.
21. Tishler PV, Larkin EK, Schluchter MD, et al. Incidence of sleep-disordered breathing in an urban adult population: the relative importance of risk factors in the development of sleep-disordered breathing. JAMA 2003;289(17):2230–7.
22. Gottlieb DJ, Yenokyan G, Newman AB, et al. Prospective study of obstructive sleep apnea and incident coronary heart disease and heart failure: the Sleep Heart Health Study. Circulation 2010;122(4):352–60.
23. Somers VK, White DP, Amin R, et al. Sleep apnea and cardiovascular disease: an American Heart Association/American College of Cardiology Foundation scientific statement. Circulation 2008;118:1080–111.
24. Peppard PE, Young T, Palta M, et al. Prospective study of the association between sleep-disordered breathing and hypertension. N Engl J Med 2000;342:1378–84.
25. Redline S, Yenokyan G, Gottlieb DJ, et al. Obstructive sleep apnea and incident stroke: the Sleep Heart Health Study. Am J Respir Crit Care Med 2010;182:269–77.
26. Punjabi NM, Shahar E, Redline S, et al. Sleep-disordered breathing, glucose intolerance, and insulin resistance: the Sleep Heart Health Study. Am J Epidemiol 2004;160:521–30.
27. Jean-Louis G, Zizi F, Clark LT, et al. Obstructive sleep apnea and cardiovascular disease: role of the metabolic syndrome and its components. J Clin Sleep Med 2008;4(3):261–72.
28. Wheaton AG, Perry GS, Chapman DP, et al. Sleep disordered breathing and depression among U.S. adults: National Health and Nutrition Examination Survey, 2005-2008. Sleep 2012;35(4):461–7.

29. Yaffe K, Laffan AM, Harrison SL, et al. Sleep-disordered breathing, hypoxia, and risk of mild cognitive impairment and dementia in older women. JAMA 2011;306(6):613–9.
30. Tregear S, Reston J, Schoelles K, et al. Obstructive sleep apnea and risk of motor vehicle crash: systematic review and meta-analysis. J Clin Sleep Med 2009;5(6):573–81.
31. Vasu TS, Grewal R, Doghramji K. Obstructive sleep apnea syndrome and perioperative complications: a systematic review of the literature. J Clin Sleep Med 2012;8(2):199–207.
32. Young T, Finn L, Peppard PE, et al. Sleep disordered breathing and mortality: eighteen-year follow-up of the Wisconsin sleep cohort. Sleep 2008;31:1071–8.
33. Hauri PJ, editor. The International Classification of Sleep Disorders, 2nd edition, Diagnostic and Coding Manual. 2nd edition. Westchester (IL): American Academy of Sleep Medicine; 2005.
34. Berry RB, Budhiraja R, Gottlieb DJ, et al. Rules for scoring respiratory events in sleep: update of the 2007 AASM Manual for the Scoring of Sleep and Associated Events. Deliberations of the Sleep Apnea Definitions Task Force of the American Academy of Sleep Medicine. J Clin Sleep Med 2012;8:597–619.
35. Javaheri S, Smith J, Chung E. The prevalence and natural history of complex sleep apnea. J Clin Sleep Med 2009;5(3):205–11.
36. Hudgel DW. Mechanisms of obstructive sleep apnea. Chest 1992;101(2):541–9.
37. Punjabi NM. The epidemiology of adult obstructive sleep apnea. Proc Am Thorac Soc 2008;5(2):136–43.
38. Young T, Evans L, Finn L, et al. Estimation of the clinically diagnosed proportion of sleep apnea syndrome in middle-aged men and women. Sleep 1997;20(9):705–6.
39. Peppard PE, Young T, Palta M, et al. Longitudinal study of moderate weight change and sleep-disordered breathing. JAMA 2000;284(23):3015–21.
40. Redline S, Tishler PV, Hans MG, et al. Racial differences in sleep-disordered breathing in African-Americans and Caucasians. Am J Respir Crit Care Med 1997;155:186–92.
41. Li K, Powell NP, Kushida C, et al. A comparison of Asian and white patients with obstructive sleep apnea syndrome. Laryngoscope 1999;109:1937–40.
42. Thomson S, Morrell MJ, Cordingley JJ, et al. Ventilation is unstable during drowsiness before sleep onset. J Appl Physiol 2005;99(5):2036–44.
43. Bixler EO, Vgontzas AN, Ten Have T, et al. Effects of age on sleep apnea in men: I. Prevalence and severity. Am J Respir Crit Care Med 1998;157(1):144–8.
44. Bradley TD, Phillipson EA. Central sleep apnea. Clin Chest Med 1992;13:493–505.
45. Epstein LJ, Kristo D, Strollo PJ Jr, et al. Clinical guideline for the evaluation, management and long-term care of obstructive sleep apnea in adults. J Clin Sleep Med 2009;5:263–6.
46. Johns MW. A new method for measuring daytime sleepiness: the Epworth sleepiness scale. Sleep 1991;14:540–5.
47. Chung F, Yegneswaran B, Liao P, et al. Validation of the Berlin questionnaire and American Society of Anesthesiologists checklist as screening tools for obstructive sleep apnea in surgical patients. Anesthesiology 2008;108(5):822–30.
48. Collop NA, Anderson WM, Boehlecke B, et al. Clinical guidelines for the use of unattended portable monitors in the diagnosis of obstructive sleep apnea in adult patients. J Clin Sleep Med 2007;3(7):737–47.
49. Marín JM, Carrizo SJ, Vicente E, et al. Long-term cardiovascular outcomes in men with obstructive sleep apnoea-hypopnoea with or without treatment with continuous positive airway pressure: an observational study. Lancet 2005;365:1046–53.
50. Morgenthaler TI, Aurora RN, Brown T, et al, Standards of Practice Committee of the AASM. Practice parameters for the use of autotitrating continuous positive airway pressure devices for titrating pressures and treating adult patients with obstructive sleep apnea syndrome: an update for 2007. Sleep 2008;31(1):141–7.
51. Aurora RN, Chowdhuri S, Ramar K, et al. The treatment of central sleep apnea syndromes in adults: practice parameters with an evidence-based literature review and meta-analyses. Sleep 2012;35(1):17–40.
52. Ferguson KA, Cartwright R, Rogers R, et al. Oral appliances for snoring and obstructive sleep apnea: a review. Sleep 2006;29(2):244–62.
53. Iftikhar IH, Hays ER, Iverson MA, et al. Effect of oral appliances on blood pressure in obstructive sleep apnea: a systematic review and meta-analysis. J Clin Sleep Med 2013;9(2):165–74.
54. Berry RB, Kryger MH, Massie CA. A novel nasal expiratory positive airway pressure (EPAP) device for the treatment of obstructive sleep apnea: a randomized controlled trial. Sleep 2011;34(4):479–85.
55. Kryger MH, Berry RB, Massie CA. Long-term use of a nasal expiratory positive airway pressure (EPAP) device as a treatment for obstructive sleep apnea (OSA). J Clin Sleep Med 2011;7(5):449–53.
56. Caples SM, Rowley JA, Prinsell JR, et al. Surgical modifications of the upper airway for obstructive sleep apnea in adults: a systematic review and meta-analysis. Sleep 2010;33(10):1396–407.
57. Guilleminault C, Simmons FB, Motta J, et al. Obstructive sleep apnea syndrome and tracheostomy. Long-term follow-up experience. Arch Intern Med 1981;141(8):985–8.

58. Tuomilehto HP, Seppä JM, Partinen MM, et al. Lifestyle intervention with weight reduction: first-line treatment in mild obstructive sleep apnea. Am J Respir Crit Care Med 2009;179:320–7.
59. Greenburg DL, Lettieri CJ, Eliasson AH. Effects of surgical weight loss on measures of obstructive sleep apnea: a meta-analysis. Am J Med 2009; 122:535–42.
60. Mehta V, Vasu TS, Phillips B, et al. Obstructive sleep apnea and oxygen therapy: a systematic review of the literature and meta-analysis. J Clin Sleep Med 2013;9(3):271–9.
61. Roth T, Schwartz JR, Hirshkowitz M, et al. Evaluation of the safety of modafinil for treatment of excessive sleepiness. J Clin Sleep Med 2007;3(6):595–602.
62. Schwartz JR, Khan A, McCall WV, et al. Tolerability and efficacy of armodafinil in naïve patients with excessive sleepiness associated with obstructive sleep apnea, shift work disorder, or narcolepsy: a 12-month, open-label, flexible-dose study with an extension period. J Clin Sleep Med 2010;6(5):450–7.
63. North JB, Jennett S. Abnormal breathing patterns associated with acute brain damage. Arch Neurol 1974;31(5):338–44.
64. Bitter T, Faber L, Hering D, et al. Sleep-disordered breathing in heart failure with normal left ventricular ejection fraction. Eur Heart J 2009;11:602–8.
65. Javaheri S, Parker TJ, Liming JD, et al. Sleep apnea in 81 ambulatory male patients with stable heart failure: types and their prevalences, consequences, and presentations. Circulation 1998;97: 2154–9.
66. Hanly PJ, Zuberi-Khokhar NS. Increased mortality associated with Cheyne-Stokes respiration in patients with congestive heart failure. Am J Respir Crit Care Med 1996;153:272–6.
67. Bradley TD, Logan AG, Kimoff RJ, et al. Continuous positive airway pressure for central sleep apnea and heart failure. N Engl J Med 2005;353:2025–33.
68. Allam J, Olson E, Gay P, et al. Efficacy of adaptive servoventilation in treatment of complex and central sleep apnea syndromes. Chest 2007;132: 1839–46.
69. Mokhlesi B, Kryger MH, Grunstein RR. Assessment and management of patients with obesity hypoventilation syndrome. Proc Am Thorac Soc 2008;5(2): 218–25.
70. Bayliss DA, Millhorn DE. Central neural mechanisms of progesterone action: application to the respiratory system. J Appl Physiol 1992;73(2):393–404.
71. Berg G, Delaive K, Manfreda J, et al. The use of health-care resources in obesity-hypoventilation syndrome. Chest 2001;120(2):377–83.
72. Banerjee D, Yee BJ, Piper AJ, et al. Obesity hypoventilation syndrome: hypoxemia during continuous positive airway pressure. Chest 2007;131(6): 1678–84.
73. Berry RB, Chediak A, Brown LK, et al. Best clinical practices for the sleep center adjustment of noninvasive positive pressure ventilation (NPPV) in stable chronic alveolar hypoventilation syndromes. J Clin Sleep Med 2010;6(5):491–509.
74. Storre JH, Seuthe B, Fiechter R, et al. Average volume-assured pressure support in obesity hypoventilation: a randomized crossover trial. Chest 2006;130(3):815–21.
75. Murphy PB, Davidson C, Hind MD, et al. Volume targeted versus pressure support non-invasive ventilation in patients with super obesity and chronic respiratory failure: a randomised controlled trial. Thorax 2012;67(8):727–34.
76. Sugerman HJ, Fairman RP, Sood RK, et al. Long-term effects of gastric surgery for treating respiratory insufficiency of obesity. Am J Clin Nutr 1992; 55(2):597–601.
77. Mokhlesi B. Obesity hypoventilation syndrome: a state-of-the-art review. Respir Care 2010;55(10): 1347–62.

Restless Legs

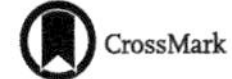

Susan Imamura, MD[a,*], Clete A. Kushida, MD, PhD[b]

KEYWORDS

- Restless legs syndrome • Clinical • Dopamine agonists

KEY POINTS

- Restless legs syndrome (RLS) is a neurologic sensorimotor disease; it is the most significant movement disorder of sleep and causes significant sleep and quality-of-life disturbances.
- RLS is a clinical diagnosis; therefore, the patient interview is sufficient in most cases to make the diagnosis.
- Behavioral interventions, such as regular exercise, maintaining good sleep hygiene, heating pads, warm or cold baths, massage, and mental distraction, can be sufficient in treating RLS symptoms, especially if symptoms are mild and/or infrequent.
- Pharmacologic interventions include dopamine agonists, anticonvulsants, opiates, sedative hypnotics, clonidine, and amantadine.

Restless legs syndrome (RLS) is a neurologic sensorimotor disease. It is the most significant movement disorder of sleep and causes significant sleep and quality of life disturbances.

CLINICAL FEATURES

RLS is a clinical diagnosis dependent on the presence of essential criteria set forth by the International Restless Legs Syndrome (IRLS)[1] Study Group, most recently updated in 2012.

The 5 essential criteria for RLS in adults are listed in **Box 1**.

Because eliciting accurate subjective descriptions of RLS sensations can be challenging in pediatric populations, diagnosis of RLS in children has the additional criteria of meeting all 5 of the IRLS criteria as well as 2 of the following 3 guidelines:

1. Showing evidence of sleep disturbance
2. Family history of RLS
3. Periodic leg movement (PLM) index greater than 5/h

RLS symptoms can be quite diverse with patients reporting symptoms of pain, aching, tingling, restlessness, cramping, pruritus, electric shocks, or crawling/creeping sensation. In addition to immobility, symptoms can be exacerbated by stress and fatigue. Although the legs are most frequently involved, RLS can also affect the arms in 14% to 50% of patients[2] and in rare cases can involve the hips, trunk, and face. Frequency of symptoms can vary from less than once a year to daily and vary in severity from mildly annoying to disabling. RLS is divided into mild, moderate, and severe categorization based on frequency and severity. Symptoms can remit for various periods of time and can be exacerbated by conditions such as pregnancy, aging, sleep deprivation as well as certain medications. Specifiers for the clinical course of RLS include chronic-persistent RLS, where the symptoms occur on average at least twice weekly for the past year, and intermittent RLS, where symptoms occur on average less than 2 times per week and with at least 5 lifetime events.[3]

Disclosure: Dr. Kushida has a research grant with Impax Laboratories.
[a] Department of Sleep Medicine, The Permanente Medical Group, 275 Hospital Parkway, Suite 425, San Jose, CA 95123, USA; [b] Department of Psychiatry and Behavioral Science, Stanford Sleep Medicine Center, 450 Broadway Street, Pavilion C, 2nd Floor, MC 5704, Redwood City, CA 94063, USA
* Corresponding author.
E-mail address: susan_imamura@yahoo.com

Sleep Med Clin 9 (2014) 513–521
http://dx.doi.org/10.1016/j.jsmc.2014.08.006
1556-407X/14/$ – see front matter

Box 1
Five essential criteria for restless legs syndrome in adults

1. An urge to move usually, but not always, accompanied by uncomfortable or unpleasant sensations in the legs
2. The urge to move the legs and accompanying unpleasant sensation is worse with inactivity or during rest
3. The urge is partially or fully alleviated by movement
4. Symptoms are worse or occur only during the evening
5. The symptoms cannot be solely accounted for by another medical or behavioral condition (eg, myalgia, venous stasis, arthritis, leg cramps, positional discomfort, or habitual foot tapping).

Most RLS cases are idiopathic or primary and these cases tend to have a familial component with rates between 18.5% and 92% of individuals with primary RLS having a positive family history.[2,4] Secondary RLS is associated with several conditions, including uremia and end-stage renal disease, iron deficiency anemia, neuropathy, pregnancy, and use of neuroleptics and antidepressants. Less commonly, secondary RLS has been associated with diabetes mellitus, folate deficiency, cobalamin deficiency, rheumatoid arthritis, fibromyalgia, Sjorgen syndrome, hypothyroidism, Parkinson disease, depression, and attention deficient hyperactivity disorder.[5–9] In comparison with primary RLS, secondary RLS starts later in life, progresses more rapidly, and tends to resolve when the underlying condition is treated. Although familial rates are lower in secondary RLS, it is still estimated that 13% of individuals have a positive family history. At the genetic level, RLS has been linked to 5 genomic loci, including chromosome 12q (RLS1)[10] with autosomal-recessive inheritance and chromosome 14q (RLS2),[11] 9p (RLS3),[12] 2q (RLS 4),[13] and 20p (RLS5).[14]

The clinical implications of RLS are significant with RLS patients reporting higher rates of daytime fatigue, unrefreshing sleep, irritability, panic disorder, generalized anxiety disorder, major depression, hypertension, and heart disease. Individuals with moderate-to-severe RLS report an average of 5.5 hours of sleep, have longer sleep latencies, and a higher arousal indexes compared with controls. RLS sufferers report reduced quality of life with up to 50% of the RLS sufferers reporting disruption of everyday activities or personal relationships. Sleep disturbances in turn lead to impaired daytime functioning.[15,16]

In terms of disease morbidity, individuals with cardiovascular and coronary artery disease were shown to have twice the incidence of RLS compared with individuals without a cardiac history.[17] Obesity, increased body mass index in early adulthood, and increased abdominal adiposity are associated with a higher likelihood of RLS, and the association remained even after controlling for variables like age, ethnicity, physical activity, smoking, and number of chronic diseases.[18] Individuals with RLS are more likely to have arthritic disease, headaches, and pain conditions.[19]

EPIDEMIOLOGY

RLS has a prevalence rate between 5% and 8.8% in adults using the minimal criteria described by the IRLS Study Group with roughly 50% of cases having infrequent or mild symptoms.[19] Prevalence of RLS in children is reported at 2%, although this is suspected to be an underestimate, with 40% of adults with RLS reporting symptoms before age 21% and 10% of adults reports symptoms before age 10.[20,21] That said, RLS is a condition where the prevalence increases with aging up to the age of 60, after which RLS prevalence may decrease slightly. Furthermore, individuals with mild or infrequent RLS may find their symptoms becoming either more severe or more frequent with age. RLS is twice more likely in women but has equal prevalence between boys and girls. Studies suggest higher rates of RLS in Northern European countries and lower prevalence rates in Asian countries, although the use of stricter RLS definitions in Asian countries may exaggerate this difference.[19] RLS can occur at any age but mean age of onset appears to range from 33 to 35 years for idiopathic or primary RLS and 42 to 52 years of age for secondary RLS.[19]

CAUSE

RLS is characterized as a disorder of the central nervous system, although the exact cause of primary RLS is unknown. Much of the hypotheses around the origins of RLS are based on the therapeutic effect of dopamine agonists on RLS symptoms and the exacerbation of these symptoms with dopamine antagonists. Furthermore, dopamine activity had circadian fluctuations with dopamine levels reaching their nadir at night and is thought to be the basis of the circadian pattern seen in RLS.[22]

On the biochemical level, increased levels of tyrosine hydroxylase, the rate limiting enzyme in dopamine synthesis, are found in the substania nigra, decreased D2 dopamine receptors in the putamen, lower dopamine levels (in the form of 3-*ortho*-methyldopa) in cerebral spinal fluid of RLS patients versus controls.[23] These findings suggest there is an upregulation in dopamine synthesis and transmission and a desensitization of the postsynaptic dopamine receptor.[24]

Further supporting the dopamine hypothesis is the role of iron deficiency in RLS. Iron is an essential cofactor for tyrosine hydroxylase and, as such, is essential for dopamine synthesis. Clinically, iron deficiency is seen in up to 31% of older individuals with RLS[25] and serum ferritin levels correlate inversely with RLS symptom severity in vulnerable individuals. Human histologic studies show markedly decreased iron and H-ferritin staining in the substania nigra of individuals with RLS versus controls.[26] In addition, nutritionally induced iron deficiency in rats results in reduction in D2 dopamine receptor bindings sites and a downregulation of dopaminergic activity similar to that seen in animals treated with dopamine antagonists.[27] These studies emphasize the interplay of iron and dopamine seen in RLS pathology.

One theory proposed by Clemens and colleagues[28] in 2006 is that RLS is caused by reduced dopaminergic A11 cells in the dorsoposterior hypothalamus. These cells are the sole source of spinal dopamine and have a presumed inhibitory modulatory effect. Hence, loss of these cells result in excitatory input for serotonergic cells to fire unchecked and result in increased motor and sensory responses. This theory has been supported by excessive locomotion seen in animal models with lesions to the A11 cells.

CLINICAL EVALUATION

RLS is a clinical diagnosis; therefore, the patient interview is sufficient in most cases to make the diagnosis. Because RLS can present as a range as physical symptoms, any description of unpleasant or restless feelings could be consistent with RLS. More important is to ask about onset and offset of symptoms. The unpleasant sensation in RLS is not continuous and fluctuates to a circadian pattern. Onset of the symptoms is often abrupt. RLS tends to be worse in evenings but can occur with prolonged periods of inactivity any time of the day. There is a somewhat protected period from 8 AM to 12 PM when symptoms are often absent or very mild and holds true even in cases of augmentation (see later discussion).

The unpleasant or restless sensations of RLS must be alleviated by movement even if only briefly. The movement in RLS is voluntary and secondary to the strong urge to move the legs. RLS may affect legs unilaterally or bilaterally and can alternate between legs but rarely affects solely one leg. Such presentation raises the question of radiculopathy.

The physical examination in primary RLS is normal, although physical examination can be helpful in detecting disorders that can cause secondary RLS or in ruling out conditions that are commonly mistaken for RLS. The differential diagnosis for RLS can be split between conditions that cause leg restlessness and those that cause leg discomfort (**Box 2**).

Differential Diagnosis for Restless Legs Syndrome

Signs of swelling, discoloration, and tenderness raise questions about vascular disease, arthritis, or trauma as the cause of leg discomfort. Findings of muscle weakness, muscle wasting, and impaired sensation are suggestive of neuropathy or radiculopathy and offer a helpful point of distinction as the discomfort caused by peripheral neuropathy overlaps with that caused by RLS. Furthermore, conditions that predispose one to RLS, such as diabetes and renal disease, also are risk factors for neuropathy.

Although RLS has no biological markers, laboratory tests can assist in ruling out causes of secondary RLS. Laboratory tests for urea and

Box 2
Conditions causing leg restlessness and conditions causing leg discomfort

Disorders of restlessness

- Neuroleptic-induced akathisia
- Positional discomfort
- Periodic limb movement disorder
- Hypnic jerks
- Propriospinal myoclonus at sleep onset
- Rhythmic movement disorder

Disorders of leg discomfort

- Peripheral neuropathy
- Nocturnal leg cramps
- Arterial or venous insufficiency
- Myopathies, arthritis
- Pruritis
- Deep vein thrombosis
- Fasciculations

creatinine can rule out uremia and end-stage renal disease. Serology for serum protein electrophoresis, antinuclear antibody, and rheumatoid factor can evaluate for rheumatologic disorders.

Because iron deficiency is the most common cause of secondary RLS, it is recommended to check ferritin, transferrin saturation, and total iron binding capacity (TIBC) levels in patients reporting RLS symptoms. Ferritin levels less than 50 μg/L warrant treatment. Ferritin is the most sensitive measure of iron stores in the body because it is the least resilient to drops in iron levels and is depleted far in advance compared with serum transferrin and hemoglobin levels. Because ferritin levels can be falsely elevated in cases of inflammation and infection, transferrin and TIBC laboratory tests can provide a reliable index of body iron stores. In cases of more pronounced iron deficiency, low iron can be detected by microcytic anemia findings on complete blood count, including low hematocrit, hemoglobin, and mean corpuscular volume. Additional useful tests include B12 and folate levels because low levels of folate and B12 can result in macrocytic anemia.

Electrodiagnostic testing with nerve conduction and electromyography is useful in ruling out subtle peripheral neuropathies.

Polysomnogram (PSG) is not typically indicated to diagnosis RLS. However, a PSG can be useful when the diagnosis of RLS is uncertain, if RLS symptoms are mild or minimal but the patient has significant sleep disturbance, or if frequent sleep disruption continues despite adequate treatment of RLS. In these cases, a PSG looks for comorbid conditions, such as obstructive sleep apnea or periodic limb movement disorder, which can exacerbate RLS. In cases where the patient has a coexisting pain disorder, a PSG can help confirm diagnosis of RLS by detection of periodic limb movements (PLMs). PLMs are seen in 80% of RLS patients. That said, a normal PLM index, especially in the context of a single study, does not exclude the diagnosis of RLS, and PSG data must be clinically correlated.

TREATMENT

Nonpharmacological Therapy

Behavioral interventions, such as regular exercise, maintaining good sleep hygiene, heating pads, warm or cold baths, massage, and mental distraction, can be sufficient in treating RLS symptoms, especially in cases where symptoms are mild and/or infrequent and should be encouraged as part of any treatment plan for RLS. Behavioral intervention can be highly effective and only about 20% of RLS cases merit pharmacologic treatment.[29]

Avoidance of alcohol, caffeine, and tobacco as well as medications that block dopamine or are centrally active antihistamines can greatly improve and potentially resolve RLS symptoms. Additional medications shown to exacerbate RLS symptoms include β-blockers, zonisamide, and methosuximide. In addition to dopamine antagonist antipsychotics (both typical and atypical), several psychotropics can exacerbate RLS, such as lithium and antidepressant treatments, including serotonin reuptake inhibitors, serotonin norepinephrine reuptake inhibitors, tricyclic antidepressants, and mirtazapine. Among antidepressants, bupropion is a notable exception in not triggering or worsening RLS symptoms and has even been shown to reduce PLMs.[30] Among the tricyclic antidepressants, those with preferential norepinephrine uptake, such as nortriptyline, protriptyline, and desipramine, are less likely to worsen RLS symptoms.

Iron therapy

Iron therapy is not effective in non-iron-deficient individuals because of minimal gut absorption (<2%) in individuals with normal iron levels. In individuals with ferritin levels less than 50 μg/mL, oral iron therapy of 325 mg twice to 3 times daily with 100 to 200 mg of vitamin C to increase absorption is recommended. Once iron therapy is initiated, serum iron levels should be rechecked 3 to 4 months after initiation of therapy and then every 3 to 6 months until ferritin levels are greater than 50 μg/mL.[31] Effectiveness of oral iron therapy in iron-deficient individuals is investigational due to inconsistent results between different randomized controlled studies.[32,33] Intravenous iron dextan therapy is effective for secondary RLS due to end-stage renal disease and is investigational in individuals with normal renal function with documented benefit in an open-label case series.[34,35]

Pharmacologic Therapy

Dopamine agonists

Dopamine agonists are the most common and most studied treatment of RLS. Dopamine agonist therapy can cause short-term adverse effects, such as nausea, emesis, somnolence, and fatigue. One of the most concerning adverse effects of dopamine agonist therapy is augmentation, whereby symptoms appear earlier in the day, with greater intensity, involve more areas of the body, or have a shorter latency during inactivity. Symptoms tend to be worse than pretreatment levels and occur earlier in the evening or late afternoon compared with pretreatment onset. Rates of augmentation increase with higher doses and longer treatment times. Because RLS symptoms can vary day to day, augmentation symptoms must be present 5 out of 7 days. The cause of augmentation is unknown, but it is thought that dopamine medication can overstimulate brain or spinal dopamine receptors, resulting in more of the drug to achieve symptom relief.[36]

Levodopa has been found to be very effective in reducing RLS symptoms but has a high risk of augmentation (71%–82%) even after periods as short as 1 month. Given the immediacy of its effect, it has been proposed as an intermittent treatment for RLS but should not be used more than once a week.

Pergolide, cabergoline, and dihydroergocryptine are ergot derivatives that are predominantly D2 receptor agonists and partial or complete D1 agonists. Pergolide is a documented effective treatment for RLS, has low rates of augmentation, and in addition, has the safest pregnancy rating of the pharmacologic RLS treatments. Cabergoline has the longest half-life of the dopamine agonists at 65 hours and has the clinical advantage of being active for 24 hours. It is the only dopamine agonist studied against levodopa in a large controlled trial and found to have both increased efficacy and lower risk of augmentation compared with levodopa with augmentation seen in 2% to 9% of individuals treated on cabergoline. However, both pergolide and cabergoline are unfavored as first-line treatments because of rare potential side effects of pleuropulmonary fibrosis and valvular disease, which is also true for all the ergot derivatives.[37]

The side effects of ergot derivates have increased the preference for non-ergotamine dopamine agonists as first-line treatment for RLS. Non-ergotamine dopamine agonists include ropinerole, pramipexole, piribedil, and talipexole. They have affinity for the D3 receptor and no effect on the D1 receptor. Unlike ergot derivatives, they are not associated with valvular disease, pleural effusions, or pulmonary infiltrates. Ropinerole and pramipexole are the most commonly used in RLS treatment and the most supported. Both have been shown repeatedly to reduce RLS severity and improve sleep quality. The optimal dose of pramipexole is typically between 0.125 and 0.75 mg every night at bedtime and has a half-life of 8 to 12 hours. Therapeutic effect remains intact 7.8 months after initiation of treatment. Augmentation has been reported in 7% to 30% of patients on pramipexole after 2 years.[38] Ropinerole is recommended at 0.25 to 4 mg with a half-life of 6 hours. Therapeutic effect remains 12 months after initiation of treatment.[39] Augmentation risk is not specifically known, although some studies have reported it as lower than pramipexole.[40]

Anticonvulsants

α-2-δ ligand α-2-δ Ligands include gabapentin, pregabalin, and gabapentin enacarbil, a prodrug to gabapentin. Both gabapentin and gabapentin enacarbil have been shown to have similar efficacy rates as dopamine agonists in treating RLS symptoms. Gabapentin is dosed at 300 to 2400 mg split between daily to three times a day dosing because of its variable half-life, while gabapentin enacarbil requires only a daily dose between 600 and 1200 mg.[41] Pregabalin can also be dosed once daily between doses of 50 and 300 mg, although it is only approved for pain at this time because there are no studies yet that have looked at the use in RLS treatment.[42] Short-term adverse effects include somnolence, unsteadiness, dizziness, and dry mouth. Of these 3 medications, only gabapentin enacarbil has been approved by the US Food and Drug Administration for specific use in RLS and is considered a first-line treatment.

Carbamazepine has been studied as a treatment for RLS at doses of 100 to 300 mg daily, but the quality of the studies is lacking because the studies predate validated measurements for and a fully formulated definition of RLS. In addition, the potential for serious side effects including liver toxicity and leukopenia make carbamazepine less attractive compared with better studied alternative RLS treatments.

Opiates

Although studies looking at the effectiveness of opiates are insufficient and its use in RLS remains off-label in all countries, 85% to 90% of patients with RLS respond well to opiates, and the effectiveness of this family of medication in alleviating RLS symptoms traces back to the 17th century for symptoms that closely resemble descriptions of RLS.[43] Given concerns for the addiction potential of opiates, it is important to identify the lowest therapeutic dose needed to alleviate RLS symptoms and screen for prior addiction or substance abuse history. Using this precaution, patients have been found to tolerate opioid therapy as a long-term treatment for RLS.[44]

Tramadol, a low-potency opioid, has been shown anecdotally to treat RLS symptoms at doses of 50 to 100 mg every 4 to 6 hours or 100 to 300 mg daily for the extended release formulation of tramadol and is thought to have a lower (but still possible) risk for addiction compared with other opioids because of partial rather than full opioid receptor activity.

Stronger opioids like methadone and oxycodone should be reserved for severe or refractory cases. The use of oxycodone at doses of 2.5 to 25 mg and a mean dose of 15.9 mg is supported

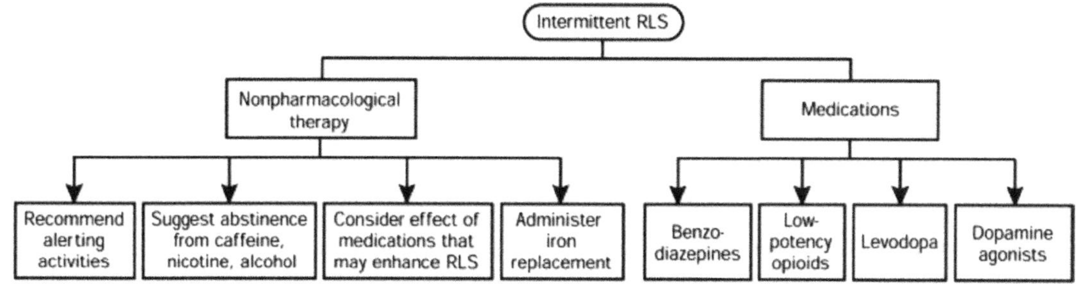

Fig. 1. Algorithm for treatment of intermittent RLS. (*From* Silber M, Ehrenberg BL, Allen RP, et al. An algorithm for the management of restless legs syndrome. Mayo Clin Proc 2004;79(7):917; with permission.)

as an efficacious treatment for RLS.[45] Methadone has been effective in RLS case studies including individuals who had failed two prior dopaminergic therapies. Methadone doses range from 5 to 30 mg daily and with therapeutic benefit lasting 6 to 12 hours.[46] Eight-five percent of patients on methadone were still on the medication after 2 to 10 years as compared with less than 20% individuals on dopamine therapy.[43]

Sedative hypnotics

Benzodiazepines and benzodiazepine-receptor agonists act on GABA-A receptor and may improve RLS by the same mechanism of gabapentin and gabapentin enacarbil. However, unlike the α-2 ligands, benzodiazepines have not been shown to reduce the PLM index. The subjective benefit of RLS symptoms is likely secondary to the sedative effect of these medications. Therapeutic response to clonazepam has been inconsistent between studies, and positive response to zolpidem is seen in one case study. Both treatments are considered investigational for RLS.[42] Benzodiazepines other than clonazepam have not been studied in controlled trials for the treatment of RLS.

Clonidine

Clonidine is an α-2 receptor agonist whose mechanism of action in RLS treatment is unknown, yet one small randomized double-blind study did show subjective improvement of RLS symptoms as well as improved sleep onset at the mean dose of 0.5 mg daily compared with placebo-treated individuals.[47]

Amantadine

In addition to its more recognized use as an inhibitor of influenza A replication, amantadine also enhances dopamine release as well as blocks dopamine reuptake, which led to one prospective study's investigation of the medication in RLS treatment. Fifty-two percent of patients of a 21-sample size had improvement of RLS symptoms on doses of 100 to 300 mg/d.[48] Given the small sample size and lack of additional supportive studies, use of amantadine in RLS treatment remains investigational. It should be used with caution in the elderly because of its extended duration of action, and reduced doses should be used in those with renal insufficiency.

Magnesium

Magnesium has been looked at as an RLS treatment in pregnant women with toxemia. In this specific group, magnesium did appear to improve RLS symptoms at a dose of 400 mg daily. It has also shown improvement in one small open study and is considered an investigational treatment for RLS.[49]

Treatment algorithms

Algorithms for treatment of RLS are shown in **Figs. 1–3**.[31]

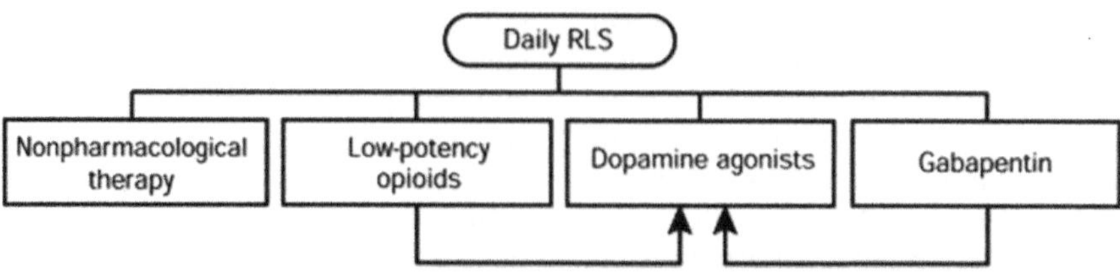

Fig. 2. Algorithm for treatment of daily RLS. (*From* Silber M, Ehrenberg BL, Allen RP, et al. An algorithm for the management of restless legs syndrome. Mayo Clin Proc 2004;79(7):919; with permission.)

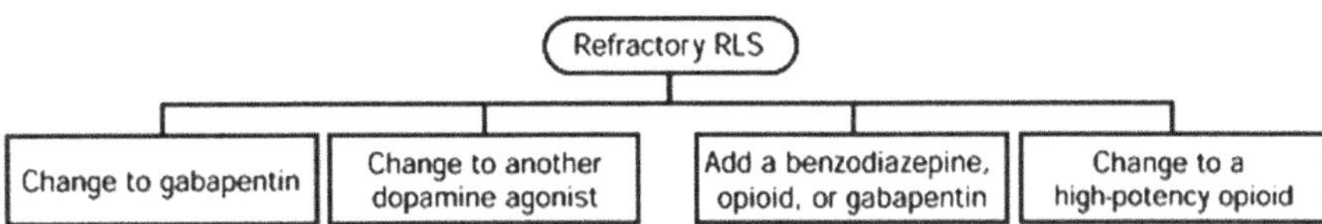

Fig. 3. Algorithm for treatment of refractory RLS. (*From* Silber M, Ehrenberg BL, Allen RP, et al. An algorithm for the management of restless legs syndrome. Mayo Clin Proc 2004;79(7):920; with permission.)

TREATMENT OF RESTLESS LEGS SYNDROME IN SPECIAL POPULATIONS

Restless Legs Syndrome Treatment in Pregnancy

RLS occurs in 20% of pregnant woman. Pregnancy increases the risk for anemia and both iron and folate deficiency should be investigated and treated if low. Behavioral management for RLS symptoms should be emphasized. Most pharmacologic treatments are category C (toxic effects in animals and unknown response in humans) or higher (known risk in humans). If RLS symptoms are severe, pergolide can be considered because it is the only RLS medication that is a category B agent (no evidence for risks in humans.)

Restless Legs Syndrome in Hemodiaylsis Patients

RLS can occur in 20% to 72% of individuals undergoing dialysis. That said, few studies have examined RLS treatment in this population group. Both levodopa and pergolide have been found to be less effective for RLS in patients on hemodialysis compared with individuals with idiopathic RLS.[50] Several case studies have reported improvement in RLS symptoms on clonidine, clonazepam, and epoetin in hemodialysis patients as well as improvement following renal transplant.[29]

REFRACTORY RESTLESS LEGS SYNDROME

Refractory RLS occurs when RLS has been treated with at least one dopamine agonist at usual doses and, unable to achieve a satisfactory response, there is a diminishing response to therapy even with increasing doses or augmentation or the individual has an intolerable adverse effect to therapy. Referral to a sleep specialist is indicated in cases of refractory RLS.

Treatment of refractory RLS, including augmentation, includes a trial with an alternative dopamine agonist because patients often show different responses to other dopamine agonists. If augmentation develops with a second agent, a switch to non-dopamine agonist therapy is mandatory. Addition of gabapentin or gabapentin enacarbil, benzodiazepines, or opioids to dopamine agonists can be effective as can a complete switch to high-potency opioids.

SUMMARY

RLS is a condition of considerable comorbidity and quality-of-life impairment that requires treatment in moderate-to-severe cases. The understanding of and treatment for the disorder continue to grow, making its clinical management an area of ongoing interest and innovative intervention.

REFERENCES

1. The International Restless Legs Study Group. 2012 Revised IRLSSG Diagnostic Criteria for RLS. Retrieved from http://irlssg.org/diagnostic-criteria/.
2. Winkelmann J, Wetter TC, Collado-Seidel V, et al. Clinical characteristics and frequency of the hereditary restless legs syndrome in a population of 300 patients. Sleep 2000;23:597–602.
3. Available at: http://irlssg.org/diagnostic-criteria. Accessed July 19, 2014.
4. Rangarajan S, Rangarajan S, D'Souza GA. Restless legs syndrome in an Indian urban population. Sleep Med 2007;9(1):88–93.
5. Wetter TC, Stiasny K, Kohnen R, et al. Polysomnographic sleep measures in patients with uremic and idiopathic restless legs syndrome. Mov Disorder 1998;13:820–4.
6. Yunus MB, Aldag JC. Restless legs syndrome and leg cramps in fibromyalgia syndrome: a controlled study. BMJ 1996;23:200–3.
7. Reynolds G, Blake DR, Pall HS, et al. Restless leg syndrome and rheumatoid arthritis. BMJ 1986;292: 659–60.
8. Picciietti DL, Underwood DJ, Farris WA, et al. Further studies on periodic limb movement disorder and restless legs syndrome in children with attention-deficit hyperactivity disorder. Mov Disorder 1999;14:1000–7.
9. Gudbjomsson B, Broman JE, Hetta J, et al. Sleep disturbances in patients with primary Sjorgen's syndrome. Br J Rheumatol 1993;32:1072–6.
10. Winkelmann J, Lichtner P, Pütz B, et al. Evidence for further genetic locus heterogeneity and confirmation of RLS-1 in restless legs syndrome. Mov Disord 2006;21:28–33.

11. Bonati MT, Ferini-Strambi L, Aridon P, et al. Autosomal dominant restless legs syndrome maps on chromosome 14q. Brain 2003;126:1485–92.
12. Chen S, Ondo WG, Rao S, et al. Genomewide linkage scan identifies a novel susceptibility locus for restless legs syndrome on chromosome 9p. Am J Hum Genet 2004;74:876–85.
13. Pichler I, Marroni F, Volpato CB, et al. Linkage analysis identifies a novel locus for restless legs syndrome on chromosome 2q in a South Tyrolean population isolate. Am J Hum Genet 2006;79: 716–23.
14. Levchenko A, Provost S, Montplaisir JY, et al. A novel autosomal dominant restless legs syndrome locus maps to chromosome 20p13. Neurology 2006;67(5):900–1.
15. Allen RP, Walters AS, Montplaisir J, et al. Restless legs syndrome prevalence and impact: REST general population study. Arch Intern Med 2005; 165(11):1286–92.
16. Garcia-Borreguero D. Time to REST: epidemiology and burden. Eur J Neurol 2006;13(Suppl 3):15–20.
17. Winkelman JW, Shahar E, Sharief I, et al. Association of restless legs syndrome and cardiovascular disease in the Sleep Heart Health Study. Neurology 2008;70:35–42.
18. Gao X, Schwarzschild MA, Wang H, et al. Obesity and restless legs syndrome in men and women. Neurology 2009;72:1255–61.
19. Ohayon MM, O'Hara R, Vitiello MV. Epidemiology of restless legs syndrome: a synthesis of the literature. Sleep Med Rev 2012;16(4):283–95.
20. Walters AS, Hickey K, Maltzman J, et al. A questionnaire study of 138 patients with restless legs syndrome: the 'Night-Walkers' survey. Neurology 1996;46(1):92–5.
21. Montplaisir J, Boucher S, Poirier G, et al. Clinical, polysomnographic and genetic characteristics of restless legs syndrome: a study of 133 patients newly diagnosed with new standard criteria. Mov Dis 1997;12:61–5.
22. Sowers JR, Vlachakis N. Circadian variations in plasma dopamine levels in man. J Endocrinol Invest 1984;7:3415.
23. Allen RP, Conner JR, Hyland K, et al. Abnormally increased CSF 3-ortho-methyldopa (3-OMD) in untreated restless legs syndrome patients indicate more severe disease and possibly abnormally increased dopamine synthesis. Sleep Med 2009; 10(1):123–8.
24. Leschziner G, Gringas P. Clinical review: restless legs syndrome. BMJ 2012;344:e3056.
25. O'Keeffe ST, Noel J, Lavan JN. Restless legs syndrome in the elderly. Postgrad Med J 1993;69: 701–3.
26. Connor JR, Boyer PJ, Menzies SL, et al. Neuropathological examination suggests impaired brain iron acquisition in restless legs syndrome. Neurology 2003;61(3):304–9.
27. Ashkenazi R, Ben-Shachar D, Youdim MB. Nutritional iron and dopamine binding sites in the rat brain. Pharmacol Biochem Behav 1982;17(Suppl 1):43–7.
28. Clemens S, Rye D, Hochman S. Restless legs syndrome: revisiting the dopamine hypothesis from the spinal cord perspective. Neurology 2006;67(1): 125–30.
29. Hening W, Allen R, Earley C, et al. The treatment of restless legs syndrome and periodic limb movement disorder: an American Academy of Sleep Medicine Review. Sleep 1999;22:970–99.
30. Nofzinger EA, Fasiczka A, Berman S, et al. Bupropion SR reduces periodic leg movements associated with arousals from sleep in depressed patients with periodic limb movement disorder. J Clin Psychiatry 2000;61:858–62.
31. Silber M, Ehrenberg BL, Allen RP, et al. An algorithm for the management of restless legs syndrome. Mayo Clin Proc 2004;79(7):916–22.
32. Davis BJ, Rajpul A, Rajpul ML, et al. A randomized, double-blind placebo-controlled trial of iron in restless legs syndrome. Eur Neurol 2000;43:70–5.
33. OKeeffe ST, Gavin K, Lavan JN. Iron status and restless legs syndrome in the elderly. Age Ageing 1994;23:200–3.
34. Sloand JA, Shelly MA, Feigin A, et al. A double-blind, placebo-controlled trial of intravenous iron dextran therapy in patients with ESRD and restless legs syndrome. Am J Kidney Dis 2004;43: 663–70.
35. Earley CJ, Heckler D, Allen RP. The treatment of restless legs syndrome with intravenous iron dextran. Sleep Med 2004;5:231–5.
36. Understanding Augmentation and Willis-Ekbom Disease/Restless Legs Syndrome: a guide to help control and manage your WED/RLS. Available at: http://www.rls.org/document.doc?id=2324. Accessed July 23, 2014.
37. Hening WA, Allen RP, Earley CJ, et al. An update on the dopaminergic treatment of restless legs syndrome and periodic limb movement disorder. Sleep 2004;27:560–83.
38. Montplasir J, Denesle R, Petit D. Pramipexole in the treatment of restless legs syndrome: a follow up study. Eur J Neurol 2000;7(Suppl 1):27–30.
39. Estvill E, de la Fuente V. The use of ropinirol ++ as a treatment for restless legs syndrome. Rev Neurol 1999;28:962–3.
40. Byrne R, Sinha S, Chaudhuri KR. Restless legs syndrome: diagnosis and review of management options. Neuropsychiatr Dis Treat 2006;2(2):155–64.
41. Brooks DJ. Dopamine agonists: their role in the treatment of Parkinson's disease. J Neurol Neurosurg Psychiatry 2000;68:685–9.

42. Trenkwalder C, Hening WA, Montagna P, et al. Treatment of restless legs syndrome: an evidence-based review and implications for clinical practice. Mov Disord 2008;23:2267–302.
43. Treatment for Restless Legs Syndrome (RLS). Available at: http://www.hopkinsmedicine.org/neurology_neurosurgery/centers_clinics/restless-legs-syndrome/what-is-rls/treatment.html. Accessed July 27, 2014.
44. Walters AS, Winkelmann J, Trenkwalder C, et al. Long term follow up on restless legs syndrome patients treated with opioids. Mov Disord 2001;16:1105–9.
45. Walters AS, Wagner ML, Hening WA, et al. Successful treatment of the idiopathic restless legs syndrome in a randomized double blind trial of oxycodone versus placebo. Sleep 1993;16:327–32.
46. Ondo WG. Methadone for refractory restless legs syndrome. Mov Disord 2005;20(3):345–8.
47. Wagner MI, Walters AS, Coleman RG, et al. Randomized, double blind, placebo-controlled study of clonidine in restless legs syndrome. Sleep 1996;19:52–8.
48. Evidente VG, Adler CH, Caviness JN, et al. Amantadine is beneficial in restless legs syndrome. Mov Disord 2000;15:324–7.
49. Hornyak M, Voderholzer U, Hohagen F, et al. Magnesium therapy for periodic leg movements related insomnia and restless legs syndrome: an open pilot study. Sleep 1998;21:501–5.
50. Earley CJ. Restless legs syndrome. N Engl J Med 2003;348:2103–9.

Periodic or Rhythmic Movements During Sleep

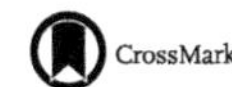

Emmanuelle Lapointe, MD[a,*], Éric Frenette, MD[b]

KEYWORDS

- Sleep-related movement disorders • Periodic limb movement • Rhythmic movement disorder
- Sleep bruxism • Hypnagogic foot tremor • Alternating leg muscle activation
- Propriospinal myoclonus

KEY POINTS

- Rhythmic movements of sleep are repetitive, stereotyped movements occurring mostly in children and usually represent a benign condition. However, other sleep-related disorders and psychiatric conditions can sometimes coexist and thus must be sought.
- Periodic limb movements of sleep increase with age and are often associated with restless legs syndrome and other sleep-related or medical disorders. Their significance is debated, but they have been associated with sleep disturbance.
- Diagnosis of sleep bruxism requires identification of tooth-grinding sounds during sleep with orodental signs or symptoms. Treatment options include occlusal splints and pharmacologic or nonpharmacologic methods.
- Hypnagogic foot tremor, alternating leg muscle activation, and propriospinal myoclonus are other rare sleep-related movement disorders.

CLINICAL CASE

John and Jane Doe, parents of John Jr, are concerned because their 2-year-old boy is having strange spells: he goes on all fours and rocks his body to and fro for about 1 minute and then falls asleep. He sometimes wakes up and then does it again and falls back asleep. He has no clear knowledge of his nighttime antics. The parents were not overly concerned until John Jr fell out of bed and banged his head during one episode. Jane has read about epilepsy and wonders whether there is a more ominous problem lurking around the corner. Otherwise, John Jr is in good health, and was born at term without any particular problem. He is doing fine in daycare and achieved all his milestones at the proper time. The parents want to be reassured and wonder whether further investigation is required.

SLEEP-RELATED RHYTHMIC MOVEMENT DISORDER

Rhythmic movement disorder (RMD) is described by the International Classification of Sleep Medicine (ICDS-3) as repetitive, stereotyped, and rhythmic movements (RMs) involving large muscle groups occurring in association with sleep.[1] The movements can encompass the head, neck, trunk, limbs, or a combination of body parts, jerking at a

The authors have nothing to disclose.

[a] Department of Neurology, Centre Hospitalier Universitaire de Sherbrooke (CHUS), 3001, 12e Avenue Nord, Sherbrooke, Québec J1H 5N4, Canada; [b] Department of Neurology, Centre Hospitalier Universitaire de Sherbrooke (CHUS), Université de Sherbrooke, 3001, 12e Avenue Nord, Sherbrooke, Québec J1H 5N4, Canada
* Corresponding author.
E-mail address: emmanuelle.lapointe@usherbrooke.ca

Sleep Med Clin 9 (2014) 523–536
http://dx.doi.org/10.1016/j.jsmc.2014.08.003

frequency of 0.5 to 2 per second. One episode can last a few seconds to several minutes, but usually less than 15 minutes. Single or multiple episodes of the same or different movements can take place during the same night.[2–5] To be considered a disorder, an RM has to have a biological consequence, such as impairment in sleep or daytime functioning, or a physical injury. The diagnostic criteria of RMD are displayed in **Box 1**.

Epidemiology

RMs are most frequently seen in infancy and childhood, their appearance shadowing the milestones of psychomotor development (**Box 2**).[5–7] Some clinicians have even hypothesized that they are implicated in motor development via vestibular stimulation.[8]

Persistence of RMs into adolescence and adulthood is increasingly recognized. One study found a persistence rate of 3% of body rocking in children at 13 years of age, but other reports suggest higher rates for RMs in adult patients.[4,5] Onset in adulthood is rare, but has been reported following head trauma and herpes encephalitis.[9] However, recurrence of a previous RMD is possible in young adults.[8]

Clinical Evaluation

Most patients encountered in clinics who are diagnosed with RMD are referred either because of concerns or complaints from their parents or bed partners or for evaluation of other sleep problems. Patients are typically amnesic of the events. Moreover, RM during sleep is sometimes viewed as a physiologic phenomenon.[8] This hypothesis is based on RMs often being self-limited and happening in normal children. In general, the disorder is mild with few episodes arising occasionally during sleep. Nevertheless, severe cases with clusters of episodes on successive nights exist. Rare complications such as carotid artery dissection, cataracts, retinal detachment, head injury, and skin and soft tissue lesions have been reported, especially with head banging.[9,10] Poor sleep quality and daytime complaints, including sleepiness, tiredness, poor concentration, and morning headache are also associated with RMD.[4,11] Some of those symptoms might also be linked to psychiatric disorders. Besides psychiatric comorbidities, sleep-related disorders should also be explored when evaluating a patient with suspected RMD (**Box 3**).[2–5,12,13]

Box 1
RMD diagnostic criteria

1. The patient shows repetitive, stereotyped, and rhythmic motor behaviors involving large muscle groups.
2. The movements are predominantly sleep related, occurring near nap or bedtime, or when the individual appears drowsy or asleep.
3. The behavior results in a significant complaint as manifest by at least 1 of the following:
   - Interference with normal sleep
   - Significant impairment in daytime function
   - Self-inflicted bodily injury or likelihood of injury if preventive measures are not used
4. The RMs are not better explained by another movement disorder or epilepsy.

From American Academy of Sleep Medicine. International classification of sleep disorders. In: Sateia M, editor. Diagnostic and coding manual. 3rd edition. Darien (IL): American Academy of Sleep Medicine; 2014; with permission.

Box 2
Clinical features of RMD

- Usually starts before 18 months: prevalence 66% at 9 months, declining thereafter to 6% at 5 years[7]
- Most common[6]
  - Body rocking (19.1%)
  - Head rolling (6.3%)
  - Head banging (5.1%)
- Less common[6]
  - Body rolling
  - Leg banging
  - Leg rolling

Diagnosis

Polysomnography (PSG) can support the diagnosis of RMD. It is helpful when the diagnosis is ambiguous or based solely on clinical grounds. In addition, PSG is useful to exclude conditions that may mimic RMD. Adding a video recording can assist in improving diagnostic accuracy. If seizures are suspected, a full electroencephalography (EEG) examination can be added.

A RM episode is recognized as a transient increase in muscle tone on electromyogram (EMG) leads and as movement artifacts on the electro-oculogram and EEG. The guidelines for scoring RMD in PSG are listed in **Box 4**.[14]

Box 3
Conditions associated with RMDs

- Psychiatric disorders
  - Attention-deficit/hyperactivity disorder
  - Anxiety disorders, depression
  - Personality disorders
  - Mental retardation
  - Learning difficulties
- Sleep-related disorders
  - Obstructive sleep apnea syndrome
  - Restless leg syndrome
  - Rapid eye movement sleep behavior disorder
  - Narcolepsy[1]

Data from Refs.[2–5,12,13]

Furthermore, use of PSG validates the relation of RM to sleep. Considered in the past to originate exclusively during sleep-wake transitions, studies including PSG have documented RMs in all stages of sleep.[2–5] Patients with RMD show normal sleep architecture on PSG. Overall, there is a slight predominance of episodes in stage nonrapid eye movement (NREM) 2.[3,5] Episodes arising exclusively in rapid eye movement (REM) sleep tend to be most common in adult patients. Co-occurrence of voluntary RMs during wakefulness is present in some patients, but their incidence only in a wake state should cast doubt on the diagnosis. These voluntary phenomena support the theory of RMD as a behavioral, self-stimulating disorder. However, this hypothesis is being challenged by physiologic propositions, such as a role for a central motor pattern generator of the brainstem during sleep.[8] Genetic factors could also be determinants, as supported by the description of familial cases.[15,16]

Differential Diagnosis

Nocturnal seizures must be differentiated from RMD (**Box 5**).[1,2,4,11] Tonic or clonic movements, tongue biting, or gaze deviation suggest an epileptic origin. However, nocturnal seizures, especially frontal-lobe seizures, can be more unusual with stereotypical hyperkinetic manifestations. Other sleep-related movement disorders must also be considered.

Treatment

Because most RMDs are mild and self-limited, treatment is often not necessary. Counseling about risk of injury, particularly if violent movements are present, is mandatory. For children at risk, a protective helmet and padding of the crib should be encouraged.

Clonazepam at low doses has been shown to be effective for treating RMD in adults and in a 6-year-old boy with fragile X syndrome.[17–19] It is effective during the first nights of administration and improves quality of sleep and excessive daytime sleepiness in some individuals. Other therapies have been attempted with some efficacy and include citalopram, imipramine, hypnosis, behavioral interventions, and controlled sleep restriction.[20] Continuous positive airway pressure (CPAP) decreases RMs associated with sleep apnea.[5,21]

Box 4
PSG diagnostic criteria for RMD

- The minimum frequency is 0.5 Hz
- The maximum frequency is 2.0 Hz
- The minimum number of individual movements required to make a cluster of RMs is 4
- The minimum amplitude of an individual rhythmic burst is 2 times the background EMG activity

From Berry RB, Brooks R, Gamaldo CE et al for the American Academy of Sleep Medicine. The AASM Manual for the Scoring of Sleep and Associated Events: Rules, Terminology and Technical Specifications, Version 2.1. www.aasmnet.org, Darien, Illinois: American Academy of Sleep Medicine, 2014; with permission.

Box 5
Differential diagnosis of RMD

- Seizures
- Periodic limb movement disorder
- Sleep myoclonus
- Bruxism
- Thumb sucking
- Hypnagogic foot tremor
- Stereotypy
- Akathisia
- Tics
- Autoerotic behavior

Data from Refs.[1,2,4,11]

CLINICAL CASE (CONTINUED)

On proper investigation and medical consultation, John and Jane are happy to hear that Junior condition is benign and will probably get better with time, but Jane formulates another complaint; John seems to be repetitively kicking while he is sleeping. This pattern is driving Jane to sleep in a separate bed. John is bewildered, unaware of his particular condition.

PERIODIC LIMB MOVEMENTS

Periodic limb movements in sleep (PLMS) are repetitive movements occurring during various stages of sleep that involve one or both legs, simultaneously or in an alternate fashion, sometimes including the arms.[1] The pattern of movements is classically described as a stereotyped triple flexion resembling the Babinski response with dorsiflexion of the ankle and toes and partial flexion of the knee and hip. However, heterogeneous patterns have been reported, suggesting that the movements are more unpredictable than was previously depicted.[22,23]

Epidemiology

High-quality data regarding prevalence of PLMS are scarce. In the largest epidemiologic study, a telephone interview survey identified a prevalence of 3.9% in 18,980 subjects aged 15 to 100 years.[24] Rates of PLMS are known to increase with age. PLMS are present in 5.6% to 23% of children referred for sleep studies.[25–27] Among 100 subjects without sleep complaints, PSG has shown a PLMS index (PLMI), the number of PLMS per hour of sleep, in excess of 30 in none of the individuals less than 30 years of age, 5.2% in individuals aged from 30 to 49 years, and 29% of individuals from 50 to 74 years of age.[28] Moreover, 45% to 70% of community-dwelling elderly have a PLMI greater than 5.[29–32]

Objective Evaluation

Clinical evaluation alone is not sensitive and specific enough to diagnose PLMS, because many people are unaware of leg movements.[33] Interviewing bed partners is often more useful when inquiring about PLMS. PSG evaluation is nevertheless indispensable. Scoring criteria are listed in **Box 6**.[14] PLMS predominates in the first half of the night. They occur mostly in sleep stages NREM 1 and 2 and decrease thereafter in NREM 3 and 4 and REM.[1,28,34]

PLM on EMG study must be differentiated from other conditions. Myoclonus, hypnagogic foot tremors, and alternating leg muscle activation are briefer and do not display a periodic character.[14] Hypnic jerks occur exclusively in transitions from wake to sleep and are also shorter in duration.

Box 6
Scoring of periodic movements in sleep

- A significant leg movement event is defined by:
  1. Minimal duration of 0.5 seconds
  2. Maximal duration of 10 seconds
  3. Minimal amplitude of 8-μV increase in EMG voltage greater than the resting anterior tibialis EMG
  4. The timing of the onset of the event is the point at which minimal amplitude is reached
  5. The timing of the ending of the event is the start of a period lasting at least 0.5 -seconds during which the EMG does not exceed 2 μV greater than the EMG resting
- A periodic leg movement series is defined by:
  1. At least 4 consecutive leg movement events
  2. Minimal length between events (time between onsets of consecutives events) of 5 seconds
  3. Maximal length between events of 90 seconds
  4. Leg movements on 2 different legs separated by less than 5 seconds as counted as only 1 leg movement
- Particular circumstances:
  1. An event should not be scored if it occurs during a period from 0.5 seconds before to 0.5 seconds after an apnea or hypopnea
  2. An arousal should be considered associated with a periodic leg movement if there is less than 0.5 seconds between them, regardless of which one is first

From Berry RB, Brooks R, Gamaldo CE et al for the American Academy of Sleep Medicine. The AASM Manual for the Scoring of Sleep and Associated Events: Rules, Terminology and Technical Specifications, Version 2.1. www.aasmnet.org, Darien, Illinois: American Academy of Sleep Medicine, 2014; with permission.

Concept of Periodic Limb Movement Disorder

To diagnose a periodic limb movement disorder (PLMD), PLMS must be associated with clinically evident sleep disturbance. Nevertheless, there are controversies regarding the clinical significance of PLMS. It is recognized that PLMS are associated with arousals. It is these arousals that are postulated to be responsible for the poor sleep quality reported by some patients.[35] Some studies have identified a correlation between arousals index (PLMA) and PSG signs of sleep disturbances, such as a higher proportion of NREM sleep stages 1 and 2, a lower proportion of NREM 3 to 4 and REM, and lower sleep efficiency.[31–33] However, in these reports and others, no links between PLMA or PLMI and subjective sleep complaints or multiple sleep latency tests, an objective measure of daytime sleepiness, were found.[34,36–38] Only 2 studies yielded positive correlations: a study by Hornyak and colleagues[39] detected a weak association of PLMI with patients' perceptions of poor sleep quality, and another by Carrier and colleagues[40] revealed a small impact of PLMI on subjective sleep quality. Thus, it is possible that it is not the PLMS per se that accounts for the excessive daytime sleepiness or nonrefreshing sleep. This possibility is highlighted by the results of Karadeniz and colleagues[41] showing that 49% of arousals occur before PLMS, 31% during PLMS, and only 23% after PLMS. Hence, PLMS may be a consequence of disturbed sleep rather than its cause.

Nonetheless, physical and psychological disorders associated with PLMS should not be overlooked. Many patients with PLMS are asymptomatic but excessive daytime sleepiness, when present, can have serious adverse consequences, as reflected by an impaired performance in a simulated driving task similar to the one seen in patients with obstructive sleep apnea syndrome (OSAS).[42] Attention-deficit/hyperactivity disorder (ADHD) also seems to be more common in children with PLMS, either resulting from common pathophysiologic mechanisms, comorbid restless legs syndrome (RLS) mimicking ADHD symptoms, or disrupted sleep.[12] In contrast, arousals accompanying PLMS are associated with autonomic activation, manifested by an increase in heart rate and blood pressure.[43] Likewise, a 1.26-fold increase in cardiovascular disease was found in community-dwelling elderly men with PLMS.[44]

Diagnosis

PLMD diagnostic criteria are highlighted in **Box 7**.[1] PLMI cutoffs of 5 in children and 15 in adults are considered significant. Clinicians should bear in mind that, in patients aged 60 years or more, a PLMI higher than 5 has not been proved to be a clear marker of sleep disturbance.[30] However, the result of the PSG should be interpreted careful, because an important night-to-night intraindividual

Box 7
PLMD diagnostic criteria

1. Polysomnography demonstrates PLMS (see **Box 6**)
2. The periodic limb movement in sleep index exceeds 5 in children and 15 in adults
3. The PLMS cause clinically significant sleep disturbance or impairment in mental, physical, social, occupational, educational, behavioral, or other important areas of functioning
4. The AASM states that the presence of insomnia or hypersomnia is not sufficient for the diagnosis of PLMD. One must exclude other potential causes of insomnia or hypersomnia and establish a reasonable cause-and-effect relationship with the PLMS
5. The movements are not better explained by another sleep, medical, neurological, or mental disorder

From American Academy of Sleep Medicine. International classification of sleep disorders. In: Sateia M, editor. Diagnostic and coding manual. 3rd edition. Darien (IL): American Academy of Sleep Medicine; 2014; with permission.

variability exists and 2 or more recordings may be necessary.[35] The periodicity index (the number of intermovement intervals between 10 and 90 seconds in a consecutive sequence of 3 or more divided by the total number of intervals) may be less variable but is not currently used in practice.[45]

Periodic Limb Movement Disorder as an Exclusion Diagnosis

Care must be taken to exclude associated conditions when evaluating suspected PLMD. Up to 80% of patients with RLS display a PLMI greater than 5.[46] Moreover, 52% of children affected by PLMD and 53% of children with RLS have been found to have a family history of RLS.[47] In addition, PLMD heralds a RLS diagnosis in many children, which suggests that PLMD and RLS may be variants of the same disease.[48] A specific variant of an intron located on chromosome 6p21.2 (BTBD9), yielding a population attributable risk of RLS with PLMS of about 50%, has been identified.[49] Excessive daytime somnolence in patients with PLMS should prompt the search for narcolepsy, because 67% of narcoleptics show a PLMI greater than 5.[50] REM sleep behavior disorder (RBD) is also associated with high rates of PLMS, with 70% of patients having a PLMI greater than 10 in a study of 40 patients.[51] PLMS in patients with RBD occurs most often in REM sleep and is associated with fewer arousals, probably reflecting loss of REM atonia and an impairment of cortical reactivity.[52] PLMS are a common finding around, and especially at the end of, a sleep apnea episode. CPAP modulates PLMS, more often reducing them in mild OSAS and unmasking them in moderate to severe OSAS, leading to an increased PLMI.[53] Again, PLMS in sleep apnea may be an epiphenomenon of disturbed sleep, as it does not seem to cause additional sleepiness.[54]

Furthermore, PLMS have been associated with a variety of medical and neurologic conditions, as listed in **Box 8**.[35,55,56] Co-occurrence of conditions in which there is an iron or dopamine deficit, in addition to the responsiveness to dopaminergic agents and opiates, supports a role for decreased dopaminergic activity in their pathophysiology. In line with the association with spinal cord lesions, it also seems that EMG analysis suggests a spinal cord origin for PLMS, perhaps with a supraspinal influence.[57] In addition, several drugs, particularly psychoactive drugs, may induce PLMS. Patients taking selective serotonin reuptake inhibitors (SSRIs) and venlafaxine have been found to have a significantly higher PLMI than controls or patients on bupropion, which is the only psychoactive drug to potentially decrease PLMS.[58,59] Fluoxetine, tricyclic antidepressants, and trazodone are other reported PLMS-inducing drugs.[60] Consequently, PSG as a diagnostic mean for PLMD should not be performed while the patient is on one of those drugs. However, according to the AASM, PLMD diagnostic can still be made even if the clinican is reasonably convinced that PLMS are induced by medication.[1]

Box 8
Conditions associated with PLMS

- RLS
- Narcolepsy
- RBD
- Sleep apnea and sleep-disordered breathing
- Attention-deficit/hyperactivity disorder
- Chronic renal failure
- Chronic obstructive pulmonary disease
- Congestive heart failure
- Essential hypertension
- Drugs (mostly selective serotonin reuptake inhibitors)
- Degenerative diseases: Parkinson disease, multiple system atrophy, corticobasal degeneration
- Ischemic and hemorrhagic stroke
- Neuropathy
- Inflammatory conditions: systemic sclerosis, sarcoidosis
- Migraine
- Juvenile fibromyalgia
- Spinal cord lesions
- Posttraumatic stress disorder

Data from Refs.[35,55,56]

Treatment of Periodic Limb Movement Disorder

After evaluation and management of comorbid conditions and removal of causative agents, treatment of diagnosed PLMD can be considered. In 2012, the American Academy of Sleep Medicine (AASM) stated that there is insufficient evidence to recommend a specific pharmacologic treatment in patients with PLMD alone.[61] Few studies focus on PLMD without RLS. Thus, practical treatment is mostly derived from evidence available for RLS management (**Box 9**).[61–66]

Box 9
Treatment of PLMS/PLMD

- Pharmacologic approach
  - First line[61]
    - Pramipexole
    - Ropinirole
    - Levodopa
  - Second line[61]
    - Gabapentin
    - Pregabalin
    - Opioids
  - Miscellaneous
    - Clonazepam[62,63]
    - Melatonin[64]
    - Valproate[65]
- Nonpharmacologic approach[66]
  - Avoidance of substances
    - Alcohol
    - Caffeine
    - Nicotine
  - Cognitive behavior therapy
  - Sleep hygiene

CLINICAL CASE (CONTINUED)

John is grateful that Jane spoke up and will modify his nicotine and caffeine intake accordingly. However, he points out to Jane that she grinds her teeth while she sleeps and this really annoys him. She had noticed jaw pain and her dentist had detected some tooth wear.

BRUXISM

Bruxism is a disorder encountered by dentists as well as by sleep clinicians. In dentistry, bruxism is regarded as a parafunctional involuntary rhythmic or spasmodic grinding of teeth. However, awake and sleep bruxism must be distinguished, because their characteristics, pathophysiology, and associated conditions differ.[67] In 2005, sleep bruxism (SB) was reclassified by the AASM as a sleep-related movement disorder, characterized by jaw muscle contraction strong enough to produce a tooth-grinding noise during sleep. This article focuses on SB, which sleep clinicians encounter more frequently.

Epidemiology

SB prevalence data are mostly drawn from transversal studies evaluating self-reported bruxism with questionnaires. A recent systematic review reported an overall prevalence of 12.8% in adults, with no gender difference.[68] A clear decrease in prevalence was seen with advancing age. However, when the diagnosis was confirmed by PSG, prevalence dropped from 12.5% to 5.5%, indicating that self-reported bruxism might be an overestimate of the true prevalence of the disorder.[69] In children, a recent review showed a more variable prevalence between studies (3.5%–40.6%).[70]

Clinical Diagnosis

AASM bruxism diagnostic criteria are purely clinical and are based on the recognition of the symptoms and signs discussed later (**Box 10**).[1]

Most bruxers are unaware of their sleep-related disorder. The most common complaint is from bed partners, who notice the sound of the grinding teeth. The force generated by masseters far exceeds that of mastication, leading to a loud, unpleasant noise. Patients can present with morning jaw muscle discomfort or fatigue, jaw stiffness, or temporal headache of short duration. Although pain in the temporomandibular region can result from bruxism, its association with temporomandibular disorder is controversial, with most PSG studies showing no relation.[71–75] Hypersensitive teeth (eg, to cold), excessive teeth mobility and metallic taste are other reported symptoms.[76–78]

Box 10
Sleep bruxism diagnostic criteria

1. The presence of regular or frequent tooth grinding sounds occurring during sleep.
2. One or more of:
   - Tooth wear consistent with tooth grinding during sleep
   - Transient morning jaw muscle pain or fatigue; and/or temporal headache; and/or jaw locking upon awakening consistent with tooth grinding during sleep

From American Academy of Sleep Medicine. International classification of sleep disorders. In: Sateia M, editor. Diagnostic and coding manual. 3rd edition. Darien (IL): American Academy of Sleep Medicine; 2014; with permission.

Clinicians must also look for signs of teeth grinding. Teeth examination can reveal tooth wear and noncarious cervical defects. Dental wear is common among bruxers and is best seen in the incisor and canine regions after drying teeth with air or cotton rolls.[79] However, tooth wear is not a specific sign for bruxism, because it is influenced by many other factors, such as age, gender, enamel properties, diet, saliva production, and gastroesophageal reflux.[77] It can thus be observed in about 40% of normal individuals and, among bruxers, does not reflect bruxism severity.[76,80] Jaw muscle examination can also be useful, showing tenderness to palpation or masseter hypertrophy during clenching. Tongue indentation, gum recession, limitation of mouth opening, and occlusal trauma are other signs to seek.[76–78]

Primary and Secondary Bruxism

Different drugs, substances, sleep disorders, and movement disorders have been associated with bruxism (**Box 11**).[76,78]

When no cause is found, bruxism is said to be primary. Various pathophysiologic mechanisms have been proposed to explain SB. Contrary to earlier theories, occlusal features of dentition do not seem to influence bruxism pathogenesis.[81] Anxiety and stress, as reflected by psychiatric comorbidities, are thought to play a role in bruxism generation.[67] This hypothesis is supported by the presence of higher levels of catecholamines in sleep bruxers' urine than in the urine of controls.[82] In children, high levels of

Box 11
Main conditions associated with SB

- Drugs
  - Recreational use: alcohol, caffeine, smoking, ecstasy[88–90]
  - Medications: SSRIs, calcium channel blockers, haloperidol, lithium, chlorpromazine, methylphenidate, atomoxetine[90–92]
- Sleep-related disorders
  - Sleep-disordered breathing: obstructive sleep apnea, snoring
  - Sleep-related movement disorders: PLMD, RLS
  - Parasomnias: sleepwalking, sleep talking, night terrors, confusional arousal, enuresis, RBD
  - Sleep-related epilepsy
  - Insomnia
- Movement disorders
  - Tics, Huntington disease, oromandibular dystonia, Parkinson disease
- Psychiatric conditions
  - Dementia
  - Attention-deficit/hyperactivity disorder[93]
  - Anxiety, mania, and depression symptoms[94]

Data from Kato T, Lavigne GJ. Sleep bruxism: a sleep-related movement disorder. Sleep Med Clin 2010;5:9–35; and Carra MC, Huynh N, Lavigne G. Sleep bruxism: a comprehensive overview for the dental clinician interested in sleep medicine. Dent Clin North Am 2012;56(2):387–413.

stress and certain personality traits, such as neuroticism, have been identified as risk factors for SB.[83,84] Nevertheless, psychological factors could have a more important role in awake than in sleep bruxism.[85] A role for other neurochemicals like dopamine, gamma-aminobutyric acid, and serotonin is also put forward by some investigators, supporting a central regulation theory.[86] In addition, the influence of genetic factors, probably through polygenic traits, seems to be important in SB.[87]

Diagnostic Evaluation

Although SB diagnosis is based on clinical grounds, it can be confirmed by PSG with masseter EMG. In a clinical setting, it is mostly useful to identify associated sleep-related disorders (see **Box 11**).[76,78,88–94] Bruxism, like other sleep-related movement disorders, displays considerable intraindividual night-to-night variability.[95] Despite this, diagnosis is constant in most cases of moderate to severe SB, but more than one recording may be necessary for mild bruxers. No important first-night effect is observed.[96]

In ambulatory studies, the absence of video recording limits the discrimination between bruxism episodes and other orofacial activities detected on EMG, such as swallowing, snoring, and coughing.[97] These nonspecific movements are known to represent respectively 30% and 85% of head and neck sleep motor events in individuals with and without SB.[98]

On EMG, bruxism is detected as sustained tonic contractions or rhythmic masticatory muscle activity (RMMA). It should be kept in mind that normal individuals also display RMMA, but 7 times less frequently than sleep bruxers.[98] Criteria for SB scoring on PSG are displayed in **Box 12**.[14]

RMMA are more frequent than tonic or mixed episodes and SB occurs more frequently in sleep stage NREM 1 and 2 and in cycle 2 and 3 of sleep.[69,99] Moreover, about 75% of RMMA episodes arise in clusters, mostly during the cyclic-alternating pattern preceding REM sleep, in which SB is hypothesized to be facilitated.[99,100] About 80% of SB episodes are preceded by cortical and autonomic arousals, as manifested on EEG and by increased heart rate.[101] Despite this, few reports suggest a link between excessive sleepiness and bruxism.[88]

Box 12
SB scoring criteria

- Brief (phasic) or sustained (tonic) increases of chin EMG activity at least twice the background amplitude.
- To be scored as bruxism, phasic increases must last 0.25 to 2 seconds and occur in a regular sequence of at least 3 increases. Tonic increases must last more than 2 seconds.
- There is a period of at least 3 seconds of stable background EMG between 2 episodes of bruxism.
- A combination of PSG and audio with a minimum of 2 audible tooth-grinding episodes per night in the absence of epilepsy is necessary.

From Berry RB, Brooks R, Gamaldo CE et al for the American Academy of Sleep Medicine. The AASM Manual for the Scoring of Sleep and Associated Events: Rules, Terminology and Technical Specifications, Version 2.1. www.aasmnet.org, Darien, Illinois: American Academy of Sleep Medicine, 2014; with permission.

Differential Diagnosis

SB must be differentiated from normal orofacial activities like swallowing and coughing, and also from other motor behaviors related to sleep (**Box 13**).[1,102]

Treatment

The decision to initiate treatment is based on the desire to prevent teeth damage and relieve SB symptoms. The most widely used treatment specific for SB is occlusal splints. These splints adequately prevent tooth wear, but studies have yielded contradictory results on their effect on RMMA.[103] Other therapeutic options are listed in **Box 14**.[103–109]

CLINICAL CASE (END)

Jane went to her dentist who fitted her with an occlusal splint.

MISCELLANEOUS CONDITIONS

Hypnagogic Foot Tremor

According to ICSD-3 criteria, hypnagogic foot tremor (HFT) consists of RMs of the feet or toes PSG shows bursts of 300–700 milliseconds foot movements occuring at 0.3–4 Hz, in trains of 10–15 seconds.[1]

The condition was first described in 2 patients following head injury, but was better characterized by Wichniak and colleagues[110] in 2001. They reported a prevalence of 7.5% within a cohort of 375 patients referred to a sleep disorder center for evaluation of other disorders. The RM occurred mostly in presleep wakefulness but also in NREM stage 1 and 2, especially during arousals. About 20% of patients were aware of the movements and able voluntarily to suppress them. No sleep disturbance was attributed to the rhythmic feet movements, which were considered benign and possibly physiologic. However, some similarities with RMD were observed in that cohort and other reported cases, which led some investigators to suggest that HFT is an RMD.[111] HFT also bears similarities with alternating leg muscle activation (ALMA), described below.[1]

Box 13
SB differential diagnosis

- Faciomandibular myoclonus
- Respiratory disturbances
- RBD
- NREM parasomnias
- Orofacial dyskinesia
- Dystonia
- Tremor
- Epilepsy (temporal lobe)[102]

From American Academy of Sleep Medicine. International classification of sleep disorders. In: Sateia M, editor. Diagnostic and coding manual. 3rd edition. Darien (IL): American Academy of Sleep Medicine; 2014; with permission.

Box 14
SB therapeutic options

- General measures
  - Avoidance of risk factors
  - Avoidance of triggering drugs
  - Treat underlying condition
- Physical approach
  - Occlusal splint
  - Maxillary advancement appliance (especially when there is concomitant snoring or mild OSAS)[104]
- Behavioral approach
  - Biofeedback
  - Cognitive behavior therapy
  - Relaxation techniques
  - Hypnosis
- Pharmacologic approach
  - Clonazepam[105,106]
  - Clonidine[107]
  - Hydroxyzine[108]
  - L-Dopa[109]
  - Miscellaneous: gabapentin, botulinum toxin, buspirone, tiagabine, topiramate[90]

Data from Lobbezoo F, van der Zaag J, van Selms MK, et al. Principles for the management of bruxism. J Oral Rehabil 2008;35(7):509–23.

Alternating Leg Muscle Activation

Alternating leg muscle activation (ALMA) constitutes a polysomnographic pattern of brief activation of the tibialis anterior, repeatedly and alternately between both legs.[1] Scoring requires at least 4 alternating muscle activations, usually lasting between 0.1 and 0.5 seconds, at 0.5 to 3 Hz.[14] The initial description of ALMA suggested that this pattern was similar to human locomotion.[112] Sixteen subjects with a mean age of 41 years were included in this initial series, with only 1 being aware of the ALMA. ALMA was seen in all sleep stages, but mostly around arousals. All patients had other sleep-related disorders, with 10 displaying PLMS. However, ALMA seemed independent from PLMS. Seventy-five percent of the 16 patients were taking antidepressants, thus suggesting an effect of these drugs on ALMA. A positive effect of pramipexole has been observed in 2 patients with ALMA complaining of poor sleep.[111,113]

Propriospinal Myoclonus

Propriospinal myoclonus (PSM) describes axial flexion or infrequently extension myoclonic jerks appearing in the abdomen, trunk, or neck. PSM arises from one spinal segment and spread rostrally and caudally along a propriospinal pathway, distinguishing it from segmental myoclonus. It is characterized by worsening with lying and by a preceding premonitory sensation in more than half of patients. A positive stimulus-sensitive response to somesthetic or, less frequently, auditory stimuli is also seen.[114] The phenomenon occurs in a quasiperiodic way mostly during sleep-wake transition and occasionally during intrasleep wakefulness, causing initial or intermediate insomnia that can be severe.[115] It also seems to be suppressed with mental activation.[116]

A definite cause can be identified in approximately 20% of cases, most having spinal lesions such as cervical trauma, myelitis, or other myelopathies.[111,114] A case series of 10 patients found abnormal spinal diffusion tensor imaging results in all of them, supporting a spinal physiologic origin for PSM.[114] Nonetheless, it has been found that PSM EMG patterns can be mimicked voluntarily[117] and a psychogenic cause for PSM has been suggested. In line with this hypothesis, a case series indicated that clinical clues suggesting a psychogenic origin, such as a Bereitschaftspotential, were present in most if not all of these patients.[118,119] Cases of PSM have also been reported following use of cannabis, ciprofloxacin, and interferon-alfa.[111]

Regarding treatment, clonazepam is the most widely used agent and has a positive effect in up to 75% of patients. Zonisamide, valproate, carbamazepine, and baclofen are other potentially effective drugs.[114]

REFERENCES

1. American Academy of Sleep Medicine. International classification of sleep disorders, 3rd edition. Darien, IL: American Academy of Sleep Medicine; 2014.
2. Dyken ME, Lin-Dyken DC, Yamada T. Diagnosing rhythmic movement disorder with video-polysomnography. Pediatr Neurol 1997;16(1):37–41.
3. Kohyama J, Matsukura F, Kimura K, et al. Rhythmic movement disorder: polysomnographic study and summary of reported cases. Brain Dev 2002; 24(1):33–8.
4. Stepanova I, Nevsimalova S, Hanusova J. Rhythmic movement disorder in sleep persisting into childhood and adulthood. Sleep 2005;28(7):851–7.
5. Mayer G, Wilde-Frenz J, Kurella B. Sleep related rhythmic movement disorder revisited. J Sleep Res 2007;16(1):110–6.
6. Sallustro F, Atwell CW. Body rocking, head banging, and head rolling in normal children. J Pediatr 1978;93(4):704–8.
7. Klackenberg G. A prospective longitudinal study of children. Data on psychic health and development up to 8 years of age. Acta Paediatr Scand Suppl 1971;224:74–83.
8. Manni R, Terzaghi M. Rhythmic movements during sleep: a physiological and pathological profile. Neurol Sci 2005;26(Suppl 3):s181–5.
9. Hoban TF. Rhythmic movement disorder in children. CNS Spectr 2003;8(2):135–8.
10. Vetrugno R, Montagna P. Sleep-to-wake transition movement disorders. Sleep Med 2011;12(Suppl 2): S11–6.
11. Khan A, Auger RR, Kushida CA, et al. Rhythmic movement disorder. Sleep Med 2008;9(3):329–30.
12. Walters AS, Silvestri R, Zucconi M, et al. Review of the possible relationship and hypothetical links between attention deficit hyperactivity disorder (ADHD) and the simple sleep related movement disorders, parasomnias, hypersomnias, and circadian rhythm disorders. J Clin Sleep Med 2008;4(6):591–600.
13. Newell KM, Incledon T, Bodfish JW, et al. Variability of stereotypic body-rocking in adults with mental retardation. Am J Ment Retard 1999;104(3):279–88.
14. Berry RB, Brooks R, Gamaldo CE et al for the American Academy of Sleep Medicine. The AASM Manual for the Scoring of Sleep and Associated Events: Rules, Terminology and Technical Specifications, Version 2.1. www.aasmnet.org, Darien, Illinois: American Academy of Sleep Medicine, 2014.
15. Bonakis A, Kritikou I, Vagiakis E, et al. A familial case of sleep rhythmic movement disorder persistent into adulthood; approach to pathophysiology. Mov Disord 2011;26(9):1769–71.
16. Attarian H, Ward N, Schuman C. A multigenerational family with persistent sleep related rhythmic movement disorder (RMD) and insomnia. J Clin Sleep Med 2009;5(6):571–2.
17. Merlino G, Serafini A, Dolso P, et al. Association of body rolling, leg rolling, and rhythmic feet movements in a young adult: a video-polysomnographic

study performed before and after one night of clonazepam. Mov Disord 2008;23(4):602–7.
18. Chisholm T, Morehouse RL. Adult headbanging: sleep studies and treatment. Sleep 1996;19(4): 343–6.
19. Manni R, Tartara A. Clonazepam treatment of rhythmic movement disorders. Sleep 1997;20(9):812.
20. Etzioni T, Katz N, Hering E, et al. Controlled sleep restriction for rhythmic movement disorder. J Pediatr 2005;147(3):393–5.
21. Chirakalwasan N, Hassan F, Kaplish N, et al. Near resolution of sleep related rhythmic movement disorder after CPAP for OSA. Sleep Med 2009;10(4): 497–500.
22. Provini F, Vetrugno R, Meletti S, et al. Motor pattern of periodic limb movements during sleep. Neurology 2001;57(2):300–4.
23. de Weerd AW, Rijsman RM, Brinkley A. Activity patterns of leg muscles in periodic limb movement disorder. J Neurol Neurosurg Psychiatry 2004; 75(2):317–9.
24. Ohayon MM, Roth T. Prevalence of restless legs syndrome and periodic limb movement disorder in the general population. J Psychosom Res 2002;53(1):547–54.
25. Kirk VG, Bohn S. Periodic limb movements in children: prevalence in a referred population. Sleep 2004;27(2):313–5.
26. Martinez S, Guilleminault C. Periodic leg movements in prepubertal children with sleep disturbance. Dev Med Child Neurol 2004;46(11): 765–70.
27. Crabtree VM, Ivanenko A, O'Brien LM, et al. Periodic limb movement disorder of sleep in children. J Sleep Res 2003;12(1):73–81.
28. Bixler EO, Kales A, Vela-Bueno A, et al. Nocturnal myoclonus and nocturnal myoclonic activity in the normal population. Res Commun Chem Pathol Pharmacol 1982;36(1):129–40.
29. Ancoli-Israel S, Kripke DF, Klauber MR, et al. Periodic limb movements in sleep in community-dwelling elderly. Sleep 1991;14(6):496–500.
30. Dickel MJ, Mosko SS. Morbidity cut-offs for sleep apnea and periodic leg movements in predicting subjective complaints in seniors. Sleep 1990; 13(2):155–66.
31. Claman DM, Redline S, Blackwell T, et al. Prevalence and correlates of periodic limb movements in older women. J Clin Sleep Med 2006;2(4): 438–45.
32. Claman DM, Ewing SK, Redline S, et al. Periodic leg movements are associated with reduced sleep quality in older men: the MrOS Sleep Study. J Clin Sleep Med 2013;9(11):1109–17.
33. Hilbert J, Mohsenin V. Can periodic limb movement disorder be diagnosed without polysomnography? A case-control study. Sleep Med 2003;4(1):35–41.
34. Karadeniz D, Ondze B, Besset A, et al. Are periodic leg movements during sleep (PLMS) responsible for sleep disruption in insomnia patients? Eur J Neurol 2000;7(3):331–6.
35. Hornyak M, Kopasz M, Feige B, et al. Variability of periodic leg movements in various sleep disorders: implications for clinical and pathophysiologic studies. Sleep 2005;28(3):331–5.
36. Mendelson WB. Are periodic leg movements associated with clinical sleep disturbance? Sleep 1996; 19(3):219–23.
37. Youngstedt SD, Kripke DF, Klauber MR, et al. Periodic leg movements during sleep and sleep disturbances in elders. J Gerontol A Biol Sci Med Sci 1998;53(5):M391–4.
38. Nicolas A, Lespérance P, Montplaisir J. Is excessive daytime sleepiness with periodic leg movements during sleep a specific diagnostic category? Eur Neurol 1998;40(1):22–6.
39. Hornyak M, Riemann D, Voderholzer U. Do periodic leg movements influence patients' perception of sleep quality? Sleep Med 2004;5(6):597–600.
40. Carrier J, Frenette S, Montplaisir J, et al. Effects of periodic leg movements during sleep in middle-aged subjects without sleep complaints. Mov Disord 2005;20(9):1127–32.
41. Karadeniz D, Ondze B, Besset A, et al. EEG arousals and awakenings in relation with periodic leg movements during sleep. J Sleep Res 2000; 9(3):273–7.
42. Gieteling EW, Bakker MS, Hoekema A, et al. Impaired driving simulation in patients with periodic limb movement disorder and patients with obstructive sleep apnea syndrome. Sleep Med 2012;13(5):517–23.
43. Cuellar NG. The effects of periodic limb movements in sleep (PLMS) on cardiovascular disease. Heart Lung 2013;42(5):353–60.
44. Koo BB, Blackwell T, Ancoli-Israel S, et al. Association of incident cardiovascular disease with periodic limb movements during sleep in older men: outcomes of sleep disorders in older men (MrOS) study. Circulation 2011;124(11):1223–31.
45. Ferri R, Fulda S, Manconi M, et al. Night-to-night variability of periodic leg movements during sleep in restless legs syndrome and periodic limb movement disorder: comparison between the periodicity index and the PLMS index. Sleep Med 2013;14(3):293–6.
46. Montplaisir J, Boucher S, Poirier G, et al. Clinical, polysomnographic, and genetic characteristics of restless legs syndrome: a study of 133 patients diagnosed with new standard criteria. Mov Disord 1997;12(1):61–5.
47. Picchietti DL, Rajendran RR, Wilson MP, et al. Pediatric restless legs syndrome and periodic limb movement disorder: parent-child pairs. Sleep Med 2009;10(8):925–31.

48. Picchietti DL, Stevens HE. Early manifestations of restless legs syndrome in childhood and adolescence. Sleep Med 2008;9(7):770–81.
49. Stefansson H, Rye DB, Hicks A, et al. A genetic risk factor for periodic limb movements in sleep. N Engl J Med 2007;357(7):639–47.
50. Dauvilliers Y, Pennestri MH, Petit D, et al. Periodic leg movements during sleep and wakefulness in narcolepsy. J Sleep Res 2007;16(3):333–9.
51. Fantini ML, Michaud M, Gosselin N, et al. Periodic leg movements in REM sleep behavior disorder and related autonomic and EEG activation. Neurology 2002;59(12):1889–94.
52. Sasai T, Inoue Y, Matsuura M. Clinical significance of periodic leg movements during sleep in rapid eye movement sleep behavior disorder. J Neurol 2011;258(11):1971–8.
53. Baran AS, Richert AC, Douglass AB, et al. Change in periodic limb movement index during treatment of obstructive sleep apnea with continuous positive airway pressure. Sleep 2003;26(6):717–20.
54. Haba-Rubio J, Staner L, Krieger J, et al. Periodic limb movements and sleepiness in obstructive sleep apnea patients. Sleep Med 2005;6(3):225–9.
55. Charokopos N, Leotsinidis M, Pouli A, et al. Periodic limb movement during sleep and chronic obstructive pulmonary disease. Sleep Breath 2008;12(2):155–9.
56. Esposito M, Parisi P, Miano S, et al. Migraine and periodic limb movement disorders in sleep in children: a preliminary case-control study. J Headache Pain 2013;14(1):57.
57. Vetrugno R, D'Angelo R, Montagna P. Periodic limb movements in sleep and periodic limb movement disorder. Neurol Sci 2007;28(Suppl 1):S9–14.
58. Yang C, White DP, Winkelman JW. Antidepressants and periodic leg movements of sleep. Biol Psychiatry 2005;58(6):510–4.
59. Nofzinger EA, Fasiczka A, Berman S, et al. Bupropion SR reduces periodic limb movements associated with arousals from sleep in depressed patients with periodic limb movement disorder. J Clin Psychiatry 2000;61(11):858–62.
60. Hoque R, Chesson AL Jr. Pharmacologically induced/exacerbated restless legs syndrome, periodic limb movements of sleep, and REM behavior disorder/REM sleep without atonia: literature review, qualitative scoring, and comparative analysis. J Clin Sleep Med 2010;6(1):79–83.
61. Aurora RN, Kristo DA, Bista SR, et al. The treatment of restless legs syndrome and periodic limb movement disorder in adults-an update for 2012: practice parameters with an evidence-based systematic review and meta-analyses: an American Academy of Sleep Medicine Clinical Practice Guideline. Sleep 2012;35(8):1039–62.
62. Saletu M, Anderer P, Saletu-Zyhlarz G, et al. Restless legs syndrome (RLS) and periodic limb movement disorder (PLMD): acute placebo-controlled sleep laboratory studies with clonazepam. Eur Neuropsychopharmacol 2001;11(2):153–61.
63. Ohanna N, Peled R, Rubin AH, et al. Periodic leg movements in sleep: effect of clonazepam treatment. Neurology 1985;35(3):408–11.
64. Kunz D, Bes F. Exogenous melatonin in periodic limb movement disorder: an open clinical trial and a hypothesis. Sleep 2001;24(2):183–7.
65. Ehrenberg BL, Eisensehr I, Corbett KE, et al. Valproate for sleep consolidation in periodic limb movement disorder. J Clin Psychopharmacol 2000;20(5):574–8.
66. Pigeon WR, Yurcheshen M. Behavioral sleep medicine interventions for restless legs syndrome and periodic limb movement disorder. Sleep Med Clin 2009;4(4):487–94.
67. Lavigne GJ, Khoury S, Abe S, et al. Bruxism physiology and pathology: an overview for clinicians. J Oral Rehabil 2008;35(7):476–94.
68. Manfredini D, Winocur E, Guarda-Nardini L, et al. Epidemiology of bruxism in adults: a systematic review of the literature. J Orofac Pain 2013;27(2):99–110.
69. Maluly M, Andersen ML, Dal-Fabbro C, et al. Polysomnographic study of the prevalence of sleep bruxism in a population sample. J Dent Res 2013;92(7 Suppl):97S–103S.
70. Manfredini D, Restrepo C, Diaz-Serrano K, et al. Prevalence of sleep bruxism in children: a systematic review of the literature. J Oral Rehabil 2013;40(8):631–42.
71. Fernandes G, Franco AL, Siqueira JT, et al. Sleep bruxism increases the risk for painful temporomandibular disorder, depression and non-specific physical symptoms. J Oral Rehabil 2012;39(7):538–44.
72. Raphael KG, Sirois DA, Janal MN, et al. Sleep bruxism and myofascial temporomandibular disorders: a laboratory-based polysomnographic investigation. J Am Dent Assoc 2012;143(11):1223–31.
73. Rossetti LM, Rossetti PH, Conti PC, et al. Association between sleep bruxism and temporomandibular disorders: a polysomnographic pilot study. Cranio 2008;26(1):16–24.
74. Barbosa Tde S, Miyakoda LS, Pocztaruk Rde L, et al. Temporomandibular disorders and bruxism in childhood and adolescence: review of the literature. Int J Pediatr Otorhinolaryngol 2008;72(3):299–314.
75. Rossetti LM, Pereira de Araujo Cdos R, Rossetti PH, et al. Association between rhythmic masticatory muscle activity during sleep and masticatory myofascial pain: a polysomnographic study. J Orofac Pain 2008;22(3):190–200.

76. Kato T, Lavigne GJ. Sleep bruxism: a sleep-related movement disorder. Sleep Med Clin 2010;5:9–35.
77. de la Hoz-Aizpurua JL, Díaz-Alonso E, LaTouche-Arbizu R, et al. Sleep bruxism. Conceptual review and update. Med Oral Patol Oral Cir Bucal 2011; 16(2):e231–8.
78. Carra MC, Huynh N, Lavigne G. Sleep bruxism: a comprehensive overview for the dental clinician interested in sleep medicine. Dent Clin North Am 2012;56(2):387–413.
79. Johansson A, Haraldson T, Omar R, et al. A system for assessing the severity and progression of occlusal tooth wear. J Oral Rehabil 1993;20(2): 125–31.
80. Abe S, Yamaguchi T, Rompré PH, et al. Tooth wear in young subjects: a discriminator between sleep bruxers and controls? Int J Prosthodont 2009; 22(4):342–50.
81. Manfredini D, Visscher CM, Guarda-Nardini L, et al. Occlusal factors are not related to self-reported bruxism. J Orofac Pain 2012;26(3):163–7.
82. Seraidarian P, Seraidarian PI, das Neves Cavalcanti B, et al. Urinary levels of catecholamines among individuals with and without sleep bruxism. Sleep Breath 2009;13(1):85–8.
83. Serra-Negra JM, Paiva SM, Flores-Mendoza CE, et al. Association among stress, personality traits, and sleep bruxism in children. Pediatr Dent 2012; 34(2):e30–4.
84. Serra-Negra JM, Ramos-Jorge ML, Flores-Mendoza CE, et al. Influence of psychosocial factors on the development of sleep bruxism among children. Int J Paediatr Dent 2009;19(5):309–17.
85. Manfredini D, Lobbezoo F. Role of psychosocial factors in the etiology of bruxism. J Orofac Pain 2009;23(2):153–66.
86. Lavigne GJ, Kato T, Kolta A, et al. Neurobiological mechanisms involved in sleep bruxism. Crit Rev Oral Biol Med 2003;14(1):30–46.
87. Rintakoski K, Hublin C, Lobbezoo F, et al. Genetic factors account for half of the phenotypic variance in liability to sleep-related bruxism in young adults: a nationwide Finnish twin cohort study. Twin Res Hum Genet 2012;15(6):714–9.
88. Ohayon MM, Li KK, Guilleminault C. Risk factors for sleep bruxism in the general population. Chest 2001;119(1):53–61.
89. Dinis-Oliveira RJ, Caldas I, Carvalho F, et al. Bruxism after 3,4-methylenedioxymethamphetamine (ecstasy) abuse. Clin Toxicol (Phila) 2010; 48(8):863–4.
90. Winocur E, Gavish A, Voikovitch M, et al. Drugs and bruxism: a critical review. J Orofac Pain 2003;17(2): 99–111.
91. Mendhekar D, Lohia D. Worsening of bruxism with atomoxetine: a case report. World J Biol Psychiatry 2009;10(4 Pt 2):671–2.
92. Mendhekar DN, Andrade C. Bruxism arising during monotherapy with methylphenidate. J Child Adolesc Psychopharmacol 2008;18(5):537–8.
93. Silvestri R, Gagliano A, Aricò I, et al. Sleep disorders in children with attention-deficit/hyperactivity disorder (ADHD) recorded overnight by video-polysomnography. Sleep Med 2009;10(10):1132–8.
94. Manfredini D, Ciapparelli A, Dell'Osso L, et al. Mood disorders in subjects with bruxing behavior. J Dent 2005;33(6):485–90.
95. Lavigne GJ, Guitard F, Rompré PH, et al. Variability in sleep bruxism activity over time. J Sleep Res 2001;10(3):237–44.
96. Hasegawa Y, Lavigne G, Rompré P, et al. Is there a first night effect on sleep bruxism? A sleep laboratory study. J Clin Sleep Med 2013; 9(11):1139–45.
97. Yamaguchi T, Abe S, Rompré PH, et al. Comparison of ambulatory and polysomnographic recording of jaw muscle activity during sleep in normal subjects. J Oral Rehabil 2012;39(1):2–10.
98. Dutra KM, Pereira FJ Jr, Rompré PH, et al. Oro-facial activities in sleep bruxism patients and in normal subjects: a controlled polygraphic and audio-video study. J Oral Rehabil 2009;36(2):86–92.
99. Huynh N, Kato T, Rompré PH, et al. Sleep bruxism is associated to micro-arousals and an increase in cardiac sympathetic activity. J Sleep Res 2006; 15(3):339–46.
100. Carra MC, Rompré PH, Kato T, et al. Sleep bruxism and sleep arousal: an experimental challenge to assess the role of cyclic alternating pattern. J Oral Rehabil 2011;38(9):635–42.
101. Kato T, Rompré P, Montplaisir JY, et al. Sleep bruxism: an oromotor activity secondary to micro-arousal. J Dent Res 2001;80(10):1940–4.
102. Meletti S, Cantalupo G, Volpi L, et al. Rhythmic teeth grinding induced by temporal lobe seizures. Neurology 2004;62(12):2306–9.
103. Lobbezoo F, van der Zaag J, van Selms MK, et al. Principles for the management of bruxism. J Oral Rehabil 2008;35(7):509–23.
104. Landry ML, Rompré PH, Manzini C, et al. Reduction of sleep bruxism using a mandibular advancement device: an experimental controlled study. Int J Prosthodont 2006;19(6):549–56.
105. Saletu A, Parapatics S, Anderer P, et al. Controlled clinical, polysomnographic and psychometric studies on differences between sleep bruxers and controls and acute effects of clonazepam as compared with placebo. Eur Arch Psychiatry Clin Neurosci 2010;260(2):163–74.
106. Saletu A, Parapatics S, Saletu B, et al. On the pharmacotherapy of sleep bruxism: placebo-controlled polysomnographic and psychometric studies with clonazepam. Neuropsychobiology 2005;51(4): 214–25.

107. Huynh N, Lavigne GJ, Lanfranchi PA, et al. The effect of 2 sympatholytic medications–propranolol and clonidine–on sleep bruxism: experimental randomized controlled studies. Sleep 2006;29(3): 307–16.
108. Ghanizadeh A, Zare S. A preliminary randomised double-blind placebo-controlled clinical trial of hydroxyzine for treating sleep bruxism in children. J Oral Rehabil 2013;40(6):413–7.
109. Lobbezoo F, Lavigne GJ, Tanguay R, et al. The effect of catecholamine precursor L-dopa on sleep bruxism: a controlled clinical trial. Mov Disord 1997;12(1):73–8.
110. Wichniak A, Tracik F, Geisler P, et al. Rhythmic feet movements while falling asleep. Mov Disord 2001; 16(6):1164–70.
111. Merlino G, Gigli GL. Sleep-related movement disorders. Neurol Sci 2012;33(3):491–513.
112. Chervin RD, Consens FB, Kutluay E. Alternating leg muscle activation during sleep and arousals: a new sleep-related motor phenomenon? Mov Disord 2003;18(5):551–9.
113. Cosentino FI, Iero I, Lanuzza B, et al. The neurophysiology of the alternating leg muscle activation (ALMA) during sleep: study of one patient before and after treatment with pramipexole. Sleep Med 2006;7(1):63–71.
114. Roze E, Bounolleau P, Ducreux D, et al. Propriospinal myoclonus revisited: clinical, neurophysiologic, and neuroradiologic findings. Neurology 2009; 72(15):1301–9.
115. Vetrugno R, Provini F, Meletti S, et al. Propriospinal myoclonus at the sleep-wake transition: a new type of parasomnia. Sleep 2001;24(7):835–43.
116. Montagna P, Provini F, Vetrugno R. Propriospinal myoclonus at sleep onset. Neurophysiol Clin 2006;36(5–6):351–5.
117. Kang SY, Sohn YH. Electromyography patterns of propriospinal myoclonus can be mimicked voluntarily. Mov Disord 2006;21(8):1241–4.
118. Erro R, Bhatia KP, Edwards MJ, et al. Clinical diagnosis of propriospinal myoclonus is unreliable: an electrophysiologic study. Mov Disord 2013;28(13): 1868–73.
119. van der Salm SM, Koelman JH, Henneke S, et al. Axial jerks: a clinical spectrum ranging from propriospinal to psychogenic myoclonus. J Neurol 2010;257(8):1349–55.

Confusional Arousals, Sleep Terrors, and Sleepwalking

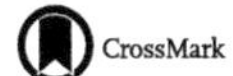

Rahul R. Modi, MS, DNB[a,b,*], Macario Camacho, MD[c], Jason Valerio, MSc, MD, FRCPC[d]

KEYWORDS

• NREM parasomnias • Disorders of arousal • Confusional arousals • Sleepwalking • Sleep terrors • Somnambulism • Pavor nocturnus • Sleep-related eating disorder

KEY POINTS

- Disorders of arousal are non–rapid eye movement (NREM) parasomnias, which share similar pathophysiology and familial and genetic patterns, along with similar priming factors.
- A detailed evaluation of the complaints along with input from the bed partner and other family members leads to a confident diagnosis.
- Video polysomnography is the investigation of choice in the case of a diagnostic dilemma. It is also helpful in identifying other comorbid sleep disorders.
- Identification and prevention of the various predisposing factors is an essential part of the management.
- Ensuring a safe sleep environment and judicious use of pharmacotherapy are cornerstones of any management strategy.

INTRODUCTION

Humans and other animals are known to exist in 3 primary states of being: wakefulness, non–rapid eye movement (NREM) sleep, and rapid eye movement (REM) sleep.[1] The sleep-wake states themselves are not mutually exclusive and exist along a spectrum of various state-determining variables. The sleep-wake states undergo frequent transitions during a regular sleep-wake cycle. This transition involves recruitment of a large number of neural networks across multiple levels of the neural axis for an accurate declaration of the state.[1–4]

This complex reorganization of the central nervous system may remain incomplete, which can lead to a dissociated state of being whereby physiologic characteristics of sleep and wake states can be identified simultaneously. Thus, an incomplete transition of NREM sleep to wakefulness may lead to a clinical scenario whereby features of both wakefulness (complex motor behaviors) and NREM sleep (lack of conscious awareness) can be seen; this is the mixed state of being. Similar mixed states of being may manifest as different parasomnias or as narcolepsy (**Fig. 1**).[1–4]

The authors have nothing to disclose.

[a] Department of Otolaryngology-Head & Neck Surgery, Bharati Vidyapeeth Deemed University Medical College, Pune, India; [b] Division of Sleep Surgery, Department of Otolaryngology-Head & Neck Surgery, Stanford University Medical Center, 801 Welch Road, Redwood City, Stanford, CA 94304, USA; [c] Sleep Surgery and Medicine Division, Department of Otolaryngology-Head and Neck Surgery, Tripler Army Medical Center, 1 Jarrett White Road, Honolulu, HI 96859, USA; [d] Division of Neurology, Department of Medicine, UBC Health Sciences Center Hospital, Suite 204, 5678 Granville Street, Vancouver, BC V6M 3C5, Canada

* Corresponding author. 670 Calderon Avenue, Apartment #3, Mountain view, CA 94041.

E-mail address: dr.rrmodi@gmail.com

Sleep Med Clin 9 (2014) 537–551

http://dx.doi.org/10.1016/j.jsmc.2014.08.009

1556-407X/14/$ – see front matter

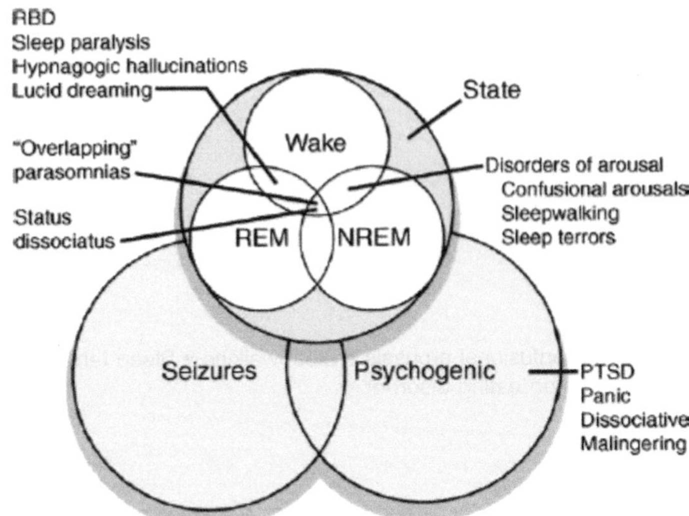

Fig. 1. The various sleep-wake disorders and relationship with parasomnias. NREM, non–rapid eye movement; PTSD, posttraumatic stress disorder; RBD, REM behavior disorders; REM, rapid eye movement. (*From* Mahowald MW, Schenck CH. Non-rapid eye movement sleep parasomnias. Neurol Clin 2005;23(4):1078; with permission.)

The recently released third edition of the *International Classification of Sleep Disorders* (ICSD-3) defines parasomnias as "undesirable physical events or experiences that occur during entry into sleep, within sleep, or during arousal from sleep."[5] These episodes commonly occur during NREM sleep, REM sleep, or during transitions to and from sleep.

This article focuses on NREM sleep parasomnias, with an emphasis on disorders of arousal, which consist of confusional arousals, sleep terrors, and sleepwalking. These conditions all result from incomplete arousals from deep sleep, and also share similar genetic patterns and pathophysiology.[5]

EPIDEMIOLOGY AND PREVALENCE

Disorders of arousal occur most commonly during childhood and become less prevalent with increasing age. Various studies have reported the prevalence of sleepwalking in children to be between 0.8% and 17%, and as high as 39.8% for sleep terrors.[6–8] The prevalence for sleepwalking peaks later around 11 to 12 years of age[7] in contrast to sleep terrors or confusional arousals, which peak in the preschool age group.[8] Traditionally considered to be uncommon in adults, sleepwalking has been reported in 0.5% to 4.0% of adults, with higher rates for young adults. The prevalence of sleep terrors in adults is between 1.0% and 2.6% and that of confusional arousals between 1.4% and 8.9%, again decreasing with increasing age.[9] Both men and women have comparable incidence, with men having a slightly higher incidence during adulthood (3.9% vs 3.1%).[10] A study on the American general population found a 29.2% lifetime prevalence of nocturnal wandering, with 3.6% of the population reporting such episodes in the previous year.[11] Overall, these studies indicate that disorders of arousal are common during childhood and are not as rare as once thought in adults.

Role of Familial Traits and Genetics in Disorders of Arousal

Genetic origins have been postulated, given the highly heritable patterns seen in NREM parasomnias. There is also genetic covariation seen in sleepwalking and sleeptalking, accounting for the co-occurrence of these disorders.[12] The largest study assessing heritability in parasomnias comes from the Finnish twin cohort study, although direct genetic analysis of parasomnias is still in its infancy.[10] Parametric linkage analysis of one family with a high prevalence of sleepwalking found possible autosomal dominant transmission, reduced penetrance, and a genetic locus on chromosome 20q12-q13.12.[13] Given that a large portion of twin pairs in the Finnish twin cohort were discordant for parasomnias, extrinsic and environmental factors are also likely to be important.

PATHOPHYSIOLOGY

Despite extensive research and the high prevalence, the pathophysiology of confusional arousals, sleepwalking, and sleep terrors is poorly understood. Most investigators agree, however, that there is a component of state dissociation resulting in sleepwalking and sleep terrors. States of sleep and wakefulness do not occur uniformly across cortical networks and are not mutually exclusive.[14,15] Electrophysiologic evidence from Terzaghi and colleagues[16] demonstrates delta bursts (representing sleep) in frontoparietal associative cortices with concurrent wake state in motor and cingulate cortices during a captured episode of confusional arousal. Functional neuroimaging, measured during a single episode of sleepwalking, demonstrated similar state dissociation with involvement of subcortical structures. Bassetti and colleagues[17] used single-photon emission computed tomography to show hyperperfusion of the cerebellum and thalamocingulate networks along with concurrent hyperperfusion of frontoparietal regions. This and other functional studies[14] support the concept of local sleep.[18] The proposed model is that in sleepwalking specific motor networks are activated and the frontoparietal and prefrontal regions are deactivated, leading to dissociation between motor behavior and higher cortical processes. Presumably this only occurs in patients predisposed to confusional arousals.

This predisposition to confusional arousals may arise from intrinsic dysfunction in slow-wave sleep in patients with a history of such events. Although there is no difference between the macrostructural sleep architecture in sleepwalkers and controls, microarousals and spontaneous arousal are more prevalent in sleepwalkers. Cyclic alternating patterns, a possible marker of arousal instability in NREM sleep, are noted to be increased in sleepwalking disorders.[19,20] Further support for a dysfunction in slow-wave sleep in patients with sleepwalking and sleep terrors derives from the altered response to sleep deprivation. Patients show both more frequent and complex parasomnias when sleep deprived but an absence of the normal rebound of slow-wave sleep seen in controls.[21] Sleep deprivation does not increase the risk of sleepwalking in control patients.[21,22]

Extrinsic factors that increase arousals from NREM sleep have also been implicated in triggering parasomnias. Sleep-disordered breathing (SDB) is the best studied trigger in both children and adults,[23,24] and treating SDB breathing can result in resolution of the parasomnia. This finding supports the notion that respiratory-induced arousals in some cases can be the cause of NREM parasomnias. Other factors that cause worsening of parasomnias are discussed in detail later in this article.

Disorders of arousal were initially thought to be an indicator of psychiatric disorders.[25–27] These patients may have a higher prevalence of depression or anxiety disorders,[9] but several studies have shown that most of these patients do not have major underlying psychopathology.[27–29]

FACTORS PRECIPITATING DISORDERS OF AROUSAL

A large number of factors (**Box 1**) have been postulated to prime or precipitate a sleepwalking episode in a genetically susceptible individual, but only a few of them have been studied in a sleep laboratory setting.[30] In general, these are factors that deepen or fragment slow-wave sleep.[22,30]

Sleep deprivation is one of the most extensively studied factors that make a genetically susceptible individual prone to sleepwalking.[22,30–35] Both partial and chronic sleep deprivation have been known to increase slow-wave sleep in control subjects, whereas in sleepwalkers an increase in the number of awakenings during slow-wave sleep and an absence of the normal rebound of slow-wave sleep has been reported.[33,35] Sleep deprivation may thus prime individuals who are genetically susceptible to sleepwalking. Pilon and colleagues[22] combined the use of 25 hours of sleep deprivation (as a priming factor) with auditory stimuli (as a precipitating factor) during slow-wave sleep to trigger episodes in known adult sleepwalkers. This study demonstrated the

Box 1
Predisposing factors for disorders of arousal

Most Potent

- Genetic predisposition
- Sleep deprivation
- Situational stress
- Forced arousal during sleep (noise, full bladder)

Other sleep disorders (SDB, PLMD)

Travel

Premenstrual period in women

Sleeping in unfamiliar surroundings

Fever

Certain medications (psychotropics, sedative/hypnotics, anticholinergics)

Abbreviations: SDB, sleep-disordered breathing; PLMD, periodic limb movement disorder.

Data from Pressman MR. Factors that predispose, prime and precipitate NREM parasomnias in adults: clinical and forensic implications. Sleep Med Rev 2007;11:5–30; and American Academy of Sleep Medicine. International classification of sleep disorders. 3rd edition. Darien (IL): American Academy of Sleep Medicine; 2014.

improved efficacy of sleep deprivation in increasing the number of experimentally induced sleepwalking episodes in comparison with normal sleep in known sleepwalkers (100% after sleep deprivation compared with 30% during normal sleep). Different durations of sleep deprivation (24–38 hours)[33,35] have been used to trigger complex behaviors in susceptible individuals.

Several psychotropic medications and their combinations have been reported to have triggered various disorders of arousal. These agents include several commonly used psychotropic drugs such as zolpidem,[36,37] used alone or in combination with other drugs, lithium,[38] triazolam,[39] and paroxetine,[40] among others.[30] A review of the existing literature on these drugs found commonalities in these reports; most of the patients on these medications had a prior history of psychiatric disorder or other complex medical issues. Only a few patients had a history of childhood sleepwalking. In most of these patients the medication was either started recently or there were increases in dosage. There was a lack of a clear, detailed sleep history, including that of other psychological stressors, in these reports. All these factors prevent formation of a clear causation between the drug and the event. There is currently a paucity of controlled studies testing the reproducibility of these adverse effects.[30]

Multiple other factors studied include psychological stress, fever,[41] pregnancy,[42,43] periodic limb movement disorder (PLMD),[30] and auditory stimuli,[22] all of which may rarely predispose a susceptible individual to a disorder of arousal. Alcohol has been thought of as a priming factor for sleepwalking events. However, with the current level of evidence it cannot be concluded that alcohol acts as a trigger or predisposes a person to sleepwalking or other disorders of arousal.[30,44]

Stronger evidence supports SDB as a trigger. Abnormal breathing events are known to cause arousals, and in individuals predisposed to sleepwalking these arousals can present as sleepwalking events because of their abnormal arousal reaction. It has been reported that in patients with sleepwalking and SDB, effective treatment of SDB alone can abolish these triggers, thus eliminating the need for additional treatment of sleepwalking.[24]

CLINICAL PRESENTATION

Because of the benign nature of these episodes, disorders of arousal may often go unreported during childhood. Presentation to the clinic typically occurs when episodes occur frequently or when violent behaviors occur. Adult patients seek treatment more often, as they are more prone to sleep-related injuries and may suffer from social inconveniences and psychological distress at presentation.[45]

These episodes commonly take place during slow-wave sleep (Stage N3), thus commonly occurring in the first third of the night. The episodes can occur at any time during NREM sleep,[2] but more rarely in N2 sleep (**Box 2**).

Confusional Arousals

Confusional arousals are also known as Elpenor syndrome after the story of Elpenor, who broke his neck during such an episode in Homer's *The Odyssey*.[27] These episodes are essentially confused awakenings whereby the patient might sit up in the bed and perform some movements with or without some vocalizations, with no ambulation. If awakened, the patient is confused and has little or no recollection of the event.[27]

Sleepwalking

Sleepwalking episodes may begin as confusional arousals or with the patient immediately leaving the bed after getting up. The patient may perform simple movements such as gesturing or pointing toward a wall, or may perform complex behaviors such as driving a car, playing a musical instrument, or dressing up. Actions lack any specific intent. Patients usually walk around with eyes open but have impaired navigation and judgment.[46] This seemingly benign condition may have violent

Box 2
Evaluation of complaints: aspects to consider

Age of onset

Evolution of symptoms

General description of events, including duration, frequency, and time of occurrence in the night

Description of the most bizarre event

Presence of recall: complete/partial/no recall

Dream enactment

Family history

Excessive daytime sleepiness

Presence of other predisposing factors (see **Box 1**)

History of injurious or violent behavior: identify the most injurious/violent behavior

History of coexisting sleep/psychiatric disorder

Medications: new medication/recent changes in dosage

outcomes with various forensic implications. Self-harm typically occurs as a result of accidental injury to the patient, and is often unnoticed until the following morning. Persons in close proximity to the sleepwalker are at a risk of injury, especially if an effort is made to forcefully curtail the activity. However, the current evidence does not suggest that these patients actively seek out and attack specific victims.[46,47] If awakened during the episode, they are disoriented and have no vivid recall of the sequence of events. This amnesia may not be complete; some patients may recall a few "images" relating to their sleepwalking activity.[21,46]

Patients who sleepwalk may also complain of excessive daytime sleepiness. More recent studies have reported 45% to 47% of patients with sleepwalking to have an Epworth Sleepiness Scale score of more than 10.[21] Another study found a significant association between sleepwalking and daytime fatigue, insomnia, and an altered quality of life.[45]

Sleep Terrors

Individuals with sleep terrors (commonly children) suddenly sit upright and emit a blood-curdling, panicky scream, accompanied by an intense activation of the autonomic nervous system including rapid breathing, sweating, flushing of the skin, mydriasis, and tachycardia. It may be an alarming situation for the parent/person witnessing the event. The individual is unresponsive and inconsolable.[2,48] These episodes resolve spontaneously in a few minutes, and the patient quickly goes back to sleep. Attempts at consoling patients may incite violent behavior and can lead to injuries to the family member or bed partner.[47] On being awakened during the event the patient is confused, disoriented, and has minimal recall of the event. Overlap or coexistence of 2 disorders does occur, albeit more rarely. For example, an episode of sleep terror may be followed by sleepwalking (**Table 1**).[27,48]

Specialized Forms of Disorders of Arousal

Sleep-related eating disorder

Sleep-related eating disorder (SRED), or sleep eating, is a disorder characterized by "recurrent episodes of dysfunctional eating that occur after an arousal during the main sleep period."[5] Other features include consumption of strange food items, sleep-related injuries, or adverse health effects of overeating.[5] The patient also has little or no awareness during the event and can injure self or others while seeking food. As with other disorders of arousal, patients typically have partial or complete amnesia after the event. The diagnostic criteria for SRED have been revised in the recently published ICSD-3 from the previous definition in ICSD-2.[5] This revision may help to differentiate it more clearly from other nocturnal eating disorders. Morning anorexia and insomnia are no longer a part of the diagnostic criteria. SRED is thus thought to be a specialized form of sleepwalking.[49,50] As with other NREM parasomnias, SRED may also be associated with PLMD and obstructive sleep apnea (OSA). Thus, sleep studies can be considered in patients presenting with SRED.[2,49,51,52] Various psychotropic medications such as sedative hypnotics, triazolam, olanzapine,[53] lithium, risperidone,[54] and zolpidem[55,56] have also been found to be associated with SRED.[49,57]

SRED may be confused with night-eating syndrome (NES), which is also characterized by excessive eating during the night. In NES, the

Table 1
Comparison of various disorders of arousal

	Confusional Arousal	Sleep Terror	Sleepwalking
Age of onset (y)	2–10	2–10	5–10
Frequency of events	3–4 per week to 1–2 per month	3–4 per week to 1–2 per month	3–4 per week to 1–2 per month
Semiological features	Sudden awakening, which may or may not be associated with vocalizations. Absence of ambulation	Screaming with intense autonomic arousal; inconsolable	Awakening with ambulation; may perform complex tasks; unresponsive to verbal commands
Time of occurrence during the night	First third	First third	First third
Duration (min)	10–30	10–20	10–20

Data from Kotagal S. Parasomnias of childhood. Curr Opin Pediatr 2008;20:659–65.

eating occurs between dinner and sleep onset (evening hyperphagia) and can be accompanied by morning anorexia and insomnia.[58] The main differentiating factor between SRED and NES is that patients with NES have awareness during the event and can recall it the following morning.[58,59] Treating isolated SRED can be challenging. Bedtime dopaminergic therapy (levodopa, pramipexole,[60] or bupropion) have been used with variable results,[49,51,52,57] while topiramate may show some benefit.[61] A randomized controlled trial is currently under way to better understand the efficacy and safety of topiramate for SRED.[62] SRED associated with sleepwalking may respond well to clonazepam and/or bromocriptine.[52] SRED associated with other conditions usually responds better when the primary sleep disorder such as OSA and restless leg syndrome (RLS)/PLMD is also treated (**Box 3**).[49]

Sleep-related abnormal sexual behaviors

A variety of sexual behaviors have been reported during sleep, in the form of isolated case reports or small case series. These behaviors are collectively known as sleep-related abnormal sexual behaviors. Other terms used to identify this condition include sleep sex, sexsomnia, and atypical sexual behavior during sleep.[5,63–65] ICSD-3[5] describes them as a subtype of confusional arousals, as the behavior is commonly confined to the bed of the patient. A classification based on pathophysiology has been proposed for these behaviors.[66] The current evidence points toward a male preponderance, with the age of onset being early adulthood.[65,66]

Clinical presentation may vary from annoying, nonharmful behaviors to violent sexual behaviors harmful to the bed partner, with possible forensic implications.[65] The symptoms reported include moaning, sexual vocalizations, masturbation, fondling, and forceful attempts at sexual intercourse. Molestation and assault on minors have also been reported.[5,64,65] A bed partner may also sustain frequent injuries (bruises, laceration) from this behavior.[67] The patients are typically amnestic of the episodes. No underlying psychopathology has been identified in these patients.[66]

Sleep sex can occur in isolation or overlap with other disorders, including other NREM parasomnias.[65] This subgroup of patients may give a

Box 3
Clinical case

A 45-year-old married woman, a housewife, was referred to our center with a history of undesirable behavior during the night by her primary care physician. According to her husband, the patient used to wake up every night within 1 to 2 hours of sleep and would head to the kitchen. She would eat small meals containing random foodstuffs such as a spoonful of salt, jalapenos, or mayonnaise.

Dream enactment was absent and the woman had no recall of these events the coming morning. This had been happening for the past 6 to 7 years. The symptoms wouldn't abate even if the patient had a snack before going to bed. The patient had recently gained weight and was worried that this habit might worsen her diabetes. Further enquiry revealed that the patient had a history of sleepwalking as a child. The sleepwalking episodes had occurred intermittently over the past 20 years. The patient had an 8-year-old son who also had history of sleepwalking.

There was no significant history of any violence or injury during sleep. There was no history of abnormal sexual behavior during sleep. Alcohol intake before bedtime used to worsen her symptoms. She denied any history of stress, sleep deprivation, or excessive daytime sleepiness. Her Epworth Sleepiness Scale score was 5/24. She had no difficulty falling asleep or going back to sleep, and felt refreshed on waking up. Snoring was present but the husband didn't witness any apneas or choking episodes. No symptoms suggestive of cataplexy, hypnagogic/hypnopompic hallucinations, or restless leg syndrome were present. There was no history of previous or current psychiatric disorder or use of any hypnotic/psychotropic medication. Physical examination was unremarkable except for a high body mass index of 36.37 kg/m^2. A sleep study done with full seizure montage showed the presence of mild obstructive sleep apnea (OSA) with an apnea-hypopnea index of 5.1, normal sleep and REM latency, and no periodic leg movements. Sleep architecture was normal with no evidence of seizure activity. No episode of sleepwalking/sleep eating occurred during the sleep study.

A diagnosis of NREM parasomnia (sleepwalking with sleep-related eating disorder [SRED]) was made. It was decided to treat her OSA in view of the concomitant history of hypertension and diabetes. A continuous positive airway pressure titration study was done and a pressure of 12 to 15 cwp was recommended. The patient was advised about proper sleep hygiene and to avoid volitional sleep deprivation. She was advised to refrain from alcohol intake. She was also started on topiramate 50 mg nightly. Significant improvement was noted in her symptoms related to SRED within 4 months of therapy.

history of previous episodes of sleepwalking or confusional arousals during childhood. The episodes may also occur as a part of REM behavior disorders (RBD),[65] parasomnia overlap disorders,[68] and nocturnal seizure disorders.[66] Patients may also have an underlying sleep disorder such as SDB, which may act as a precipitating factor, as use of continuous positive airway pressure has been shown to ameliorate the symptoms.[66] Evaluation of sleep sex involves taking a detailed sleep history and use of video polysomnography (PSG). The importance of a PSG lies in detecting the underlying disorder rather than recording the atypical behaviors, as they rarely occur in a laboratory setting.[63] Treatment of the underlying SDB, if present, is essential. Benzodiazepines, especially clonazepam, are the preferred drugs, and have shown to be highly effective in behaviors associated with NREM parasomnias and RBD.[63,67] Anticonvulsants are recommended for patients with epileptic sexsomnia.[67]

DIAGNOSIS

A systematic evaluation of the patient's complaints is the cornerstone of a successful diagnosis. The evaluation is incomplete without the history from a bed partner or a family member who has witnessed such an event. Many of these events may go unnoticed if the patient is sleeping alone. An accurate description of the event is particularly helpful, including information about awareness after the event and recall of events in the morning. Video recordings of the event at home may provide vital clues to the diagnosis.[2,69]

The diagnostic criteria mentioned in ICSD-3[5] are commonly followed to make a diagnosis of disorders of arousal. These criteria are presented in **Box 4**.

Other diagnostic criteria are suggested in the *Diagnostic and Statistical Manual of Mental Disorders*, 5th edition (DSM-5).[70] Both of these diagnostic schemas are largely in agreement for features that are essential for diagnosis. However, there are subtle differences, as follows:

1. ICSD-3 labels abnormal NREM sleep arousals under a common condition called "disorder of arousals," which is further subclassified, whereas DSM-5 does not define any such condition.
2. ICSD-3 labels arousals devoid of terror and ambulation outside of bed as confusional arousals; however, no similar condition is defined by DSM-5. Moreover, sleep-related sexual behaviors (sexsomnias) are classified as a subtype of confusional arousal in ICSD-3, whereas in DSM-5 sexsomnias are classified as a variant of sleepwalking.
3. DSM-5 identifies SRED as a subtype of sleepwalking, whereas ICSD-3 classifies it as a distinct parasomnia from the disorder of arousals.

A formal evaluation should also include a history of comorbid sleep disorders (such as OSA, RLS with PLMD), previous psychiatric history, or use of any psychotropic medications.[21,24,27] Assessment of any functional daytime impairment or excessive daytime sleepiness is also important.[45]

Box 4
ICSD-3 diagnostic criteria for disorders of arousal

General Diagnostic Criteria

A. Recurrent episodes of incomplete awakening from sleep
B. Inappropriate or absent responsiveness to efforts of others to intervene or redirect the person during the episode
C. Limited (eg, a single visual scene) or no associated cognition or dream imagery
D. Partial or complete amnesia for the episode
E. The disturbance is not better explained by another sleep disorder, mental disorder, medical condition, medication, or substance use

Sleepwalking[a]

A. The arousals are associated with ambulation and other complex behaviors out of bed

Sleep Terrors[a]

A. The arousals are characterized by episodes of abrupt terror, typically beginning with an alarming vocalization such as a frightening scream
B. There is intense fear and signs of autonomic arousal, including mydriasis, tachycardia, tachypnea, and diaphoresis during an episode

Confusional Arousals[a]

A. The episodes are characterized by mental confusion or confused behavior that occurs while the patient is in bed
B. There is an absence of terror or ambulation outside of the bed

[a] The disorder should also meet the general diagnostic criteria for NREM disorders of arousal.

From American Academy of Sleep Medicine. International classification of sleep disorders. In: Sateia M, editor. Diagnostic and coding manual. 3rd edition. Darien (IL): American Academy of Sleep Medicine; 2014; with permission.

INVESTIGATIONS

Role of Polysomnography in the Diagnosis of Disorders of Arousal

Video PSG is an expensive but useful tool in the diagnostic armamentarium for diagnosing disorders of arousal. It is not routinely indicated in uncomplicated, typical presentations with no history of violent or injurious behavior.[71]

As recommended by the American Academy of Sleep Medicine,[71] video PSG is indicated in the following scenarios.

1. Where there is confusion between the diagnosis of parasomnia or a seizure disorder
2. Where there is history of violent or potentially injurious behavior during sleep
3. Where the history is atypical in its clinical presentation (with regard to the age of onset, the time, duration or frequency of occurrence of the behavior, or presence of certain motor patterns)
4. Where the response to therapy is suboptimal

PSG is also indicated if other sleep disorders such as SDB or PLMD are thought to coexist.[24]

At present, there is a lack of consensus over the protocol considered ideal for evaluation of disorders of arousal using video PSG. A routine sleep study adds little to the diagnosis. It must be accompanied by additional electroencephalography (EEG) derivations with bilateral montage and continuous audiovisual recording.[71,72] Sphenoidal or zygomatic electrodes may also be placed to improve the sensitivity for detecting interictal EEG findings.[73] The presence of a trained technician or physician is essential for these studies to identify subtle changes in the EEG.[71,72]

A video PSG evaluation is also challenging in these patients, as episodes may not occur in the sleep laboratory.[22,74] Several modifications in the standard methodology to conduct a sleep study have been suggested to improve the efficacy of these studies, including 25 to 38 hours of sleep deprivation, the use of auditory stimuli, and recording on multiple nights.[22,35] A 2008 study[22] showed encouraging results in inducing complex behaviors during a sleep study with the use of 25 hours of sleep deprivation and timed auditory stimuli during recovery slow-wave sleep.

Electroencephalography Findings in Disorders of Arousal

EEG findings that have been shown to be commonly present in individuals with a history of disorders of arousal include increased percentage of slow-wave sleep,[75] presence of hypersynchronous delta waves,[76] and increased number of microarousals during slow-wave sleep.[74,77,78] However, none of these has been reported to have sensitivity or specificity high enough to be utilized for diagnostic purposes.[34,72] Hypersynchronous delta waves are high-amplitude delta waves observed immediately before a complex behavior or an arousal in slow-wave sleep. Studies have conducted analyses of slow-wave activity immediately before a complex behavior in the sleep laboratory to identify different markers, but have met with limited success (**Fig. 2**).[32,79]

DIFFERENTIAL DIAGNOSIS

Disorders of arousal may be confused with a variety of conditions. Confusional arousals and sleepwalking may be confused with RBD, nocturnal frontal lobe epilepsy, or psychogenic dissociative disorders. It is also important to identify malingering patients, especially in forensics cases. Sleep terrors can also be misdiagnosed as nocturnal panic attacks, nightmare disorder, or RBD (**Table 2**).[27]

RBD are characterized by sleep-related vocalization or complex motor behaviors during REM sleep,[5] with a loss of normal REM sleep atonia, thus allowing the patient to act out his or her dreams.[80,81] The episodes commonly occur in the second half of the night in contrast to disorders of arousal, which occur during the first half of the night. Multiple brief episodes may occur in the same night. The patient is generally oriented on awakening and has a clear recall of his or her dream. The sleep behavior may be violent and self-protective depending on the dream content. Dream content also changes with the development of RBD, with frightful and violent dreams occurring more frequently. Moreover, these patients typically have an older age of onset than that for disorders of arousal, and there often is no childhood or family history. In cases of doubt, video PSG can help in establishing a diagnosis by documenting a period of REM sleep without atonia.[5] These disorders are also known to be associated with several central nervous system disorders, more commonly with synucleinopathies such as multiple system atrophy, Parkinson disease, pure autonomic failure, or dementia with Lewy bodies.[82–84] However, RBD may coexist with other NREM parasomnias, such as parasomnia overlap disorder.[5,85] This disorder has an earlier age of onset than isolated RBD and has behavioral manifestations of both REM and NREM sleep parasomnias.

Seizure disorders may closely mimic disorders of arousal making the distinction difficult. Nocturnal frontal lobe epilepsy (NFLE) is a

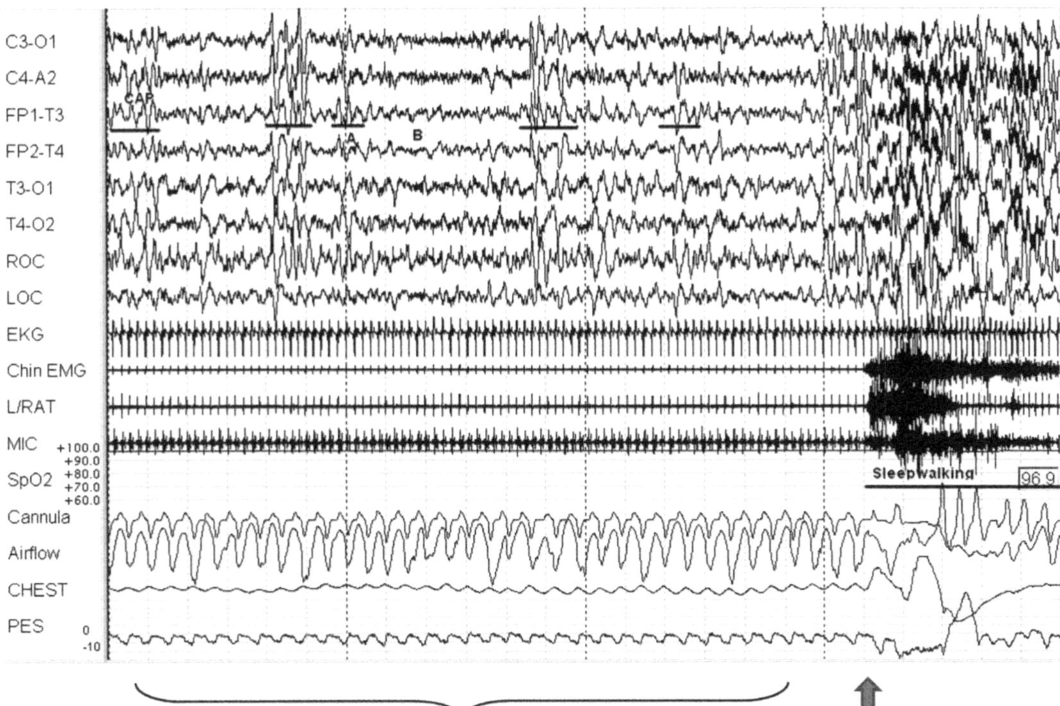

Fig. 2. Episode of sleepwalking in a child. The event begins during delta waves, as seen in the seconds just preceding beginning of movements (*arrow*). The "cyclic alternating pattern" (*downward open bracket*) is also evident on the slide. The presence of such a pattern may be associated with instability during NREM sleep. (*Courtesy of* Dr Christian Guilleminault, The Stanford Center for Sleep Sciences and Medicine, Redwood City, CA.)

syndrome characterized by occurrence of sleep-related seizures of varying complexity and duration.[86] The semiology of seizures in NFLE is highly variable, but can consist of sustained dystonic posturing and other bizarre motor behaviors occurring exclusively during sleep.[72] The episodes tend to afflict all age groups and typically occur outside of REM sleep. The motor activity can be stereotyped with dyskinetic and dystonic features, differing from the complex, more coordinated activity seen in sleepwalking or confusional arousals. The episodes are short (seconds to a few minutes), and multiple events can occur in the same night. The events can also occur during daytime napping, which would be rare for NREM parasomnias. A strong autonomic discharge is also known to occur during these seizures somewhat similar to, but less than that of sleep terrors. The patient can have complete awareness postictally with inconsistent recall of the event.[87,88] There is no dream mentation. Seizure disorders rarely undergo spontaneous remission, as opposed to the disorders of arousal, which tend to disappear with increasing age. However, differentiation solely based on history may not be possible, especially in children.[72,89] A study comparing semiologic features of NFLE and disorders of arousal found that behaviors such as standing, sitting, and walking could not be used to differentiate parasomnias from seizure disorders. Dystonic posturing and automatisms such as kicking suggested NFLE, whereas features such as failure to achieve a complete arousal suggested a diagnosis of parasomnias.[90] This study has also reported 94% success in diagnosing NFLE using a developed algorithm.

Home video recordings of the event may also help in the diagnosis of these disorders, especially with the presence of major episodes; however, lack of definite diagnostic criteria limits its use in minor attacks.[86,91–93] The current gold standard for differentiating between NFLE and NREM parasomnias is video PSG. Along with interictal EEG recordings, video analysis of semiologic features using a diagnostic algorithm may provide an answer to the diagnostic dilemma. Other approaches used to differentiate a seizure disorder from a disorder of arousal include a therapeutic trial[94] of carbamazepine in suspected seizure disorders, and the use of diagnostic scales.[93,95] Both of these approaches have had some success.

Nightmare disorder forms a major differential diagnosis for sleep terrors. This disorder is characterized by repetitive disturbing dreams that

Table 2
Differential diagnosis for disorders of arousal

	Disorders of Arousal	Nightmares	RBD	NFLE
Age of onset (y)	2–10	3–6	≥50	Any age
Gender	Either	Either	Male predominance	Male predominance
Family history of parasomnias	Present	Present	Absent	Absent
Evolution of symptoms	Tend to disappear as age increases	Tend to disappear as age increases	Rarely remit spontaneously	? Increased frequency
Overall frequency	3–4 per week to 1–2 per month	3–4 per week to 1–2 per month	Almost every night	Almost every night
Episodes/night	Usually 1	Usually 1	One to several	Several
Duration of episodes	1–10 min	3–30 min	1–2 min	Seconds to 3 min
Time of occurrence during the night	First third	Last third	At least 90 min after sleep onset	Any time
Sleep stage of onset	Slow-wave sleep (NREM)	REM sleep	REM sleep	NREM mainly stage 2
Stereotypic motor pattern	Absent	Absent	Absent	Present
Consciousness if awakened	Impaired	Normal	Normal	Normal
Recall of the episode	Absent	Present	Present	Variable

Abbreviations: NFLE, nocturnal frontal lobe epilepsy; RBD, REM behavior disorder.

Data from Kotagal S. Parasomnias of childhood. Curr Opin Pediatr 2008;20:659–65; and Tinuper P, Provini F, Bisulli F, et al. Movement disorders in sleep: guidelines for differentiating epileptic from non-epileptic motor phenomena arising from sleep. Sleep Med Rev 2007;11:255–67.

commonly cause the patient to wake up.[5] Being a REM sleep phenomenon, nightmares frequently occur during the second half of the night and are very common in childhood. The patient has a vivid recall of dreams and becomes oriented and alert immediately on waking up. In contrast to sleep terrors, these events are rarely accompanied by loud screams, and the extent of autonomic arousal (sweating, tachycardia, and palpitations) is also limited in comparison with a sleep terror. It is challenging to differentiate them in young children, from whom often a detailed history is not possible.[5,27]

Nocturnal panic attacks are common in patients with generalized panic disorders. These attacks usually occur during the N2 or N3 stage of sleep and are not accompanied by loud screaming and the intense autonomic arousal characteristic of sleep terrors.[96] Unlike in sleep terrors these patients are oriented, have a lucid recall of their dreams, and complain of difficulty falling asleep after a panic attack.

Cluster headaches in young children may be misdiagnosed as sleep terrors, and often have a dramatic response to indomethacin.[97] Other disorders reported to have an association with disorders of arousal include Tourette syndrome,[98,99] migraine,[100] and neurofibromatosis type 1.[101]

MANAGEMENT

Disorders of arousal are conditions that have an overall benign, self-limiting course. The management required for most of these individuals is accurate diagnosis and supportive care. It is important to assess the disease severity, and to identify other comorbid sleep disorders and any medications that may be responsible for precipitating this condition.[102]

Good sleep hygiene and a safe sleep environment form the cornerstone for any successful plan of management. Good sleep hygiene includes avoiding alcohol, caffeine late at night, and having a regular sleep-wake cycle.[103] It is important to avoid sleep deprivation and other stressors. Removal of firearms, knives, or any dangerous objects from the bedroom is recommended. Bolting the windows ensures safety and will prevent defenestration. More practical measures, however, may include using heavy draped curtains, or sleeping on the main level. Door alarms can be used to alert the sleepwalkers and other members in the household.[102] Caution must be exercised during the episode, and efforts to curtail the event forcefully may result in violent behavior, often more severe than expected.[47] It is also advised that these patients should sleep alone until the disorder is under control, as the bed partner is at risk of injury owing to his or her proximity.[47,102] These simple and helpful measures ensure a safe course for the disorder.

Patients who require further evaluation include those with impaired daytime performance, a history of violent or potentially injurious behavior, or unusual clinical characteristics, and those in whom events occur frequently enough to bother other family members.[2]

Confusional Arousals

It is important to reassure parents regarding the benign nature of this disorder and its self-limiting course, as most children outgrow it. Scheduled awakenings 10 to 15 minutes before the anticipated time of the arousals have been described as an effective way of controlling these episodes in children. The children are woken up and comforted by the parent. Treatment using this technique has been reported to be effective for a period of 3 to 6 months after cessation of therapy.[104]

Sleepwalking

Apart from the general measures explained earlier, other nonpharmacologic measures include use of psychotherapy, stress management,[105] and hypnotherapy.[106,107]

Pharmacotherapy is recommended for patients at risk of violent or potentially injurious behavior to self or other family members.[21] There are currently no adequately powered randomized controlled trials that have tested the efficacy of any particular drug or medication.[108] Benzodiazepines (BZDs) are the drugs commonly used for this condition. Clonazepam[103,109] at a dose of 0.5 to 1.0 mg, 30 to 60 minutes before anticipated bedtime, is usually effective; this gives the drug enough time to reach key brain sites for optimal action, as these episodes can occur as early as 15 minutes after sleep onset.[102] Other recommended drugs include diazepam[110] and triazolam.[111] Non-BZDs used for the treatment of sleepwalking include imipramine,[110] paroxetine,[112] and melatonin.[113]

Sleep Terrors

Young children with a history of infrequent episodes of sleep terror usually outgrow the disease by adolescence, so parental reassurance is typically all that is required.[114] Parents or caretakers must be informed to avoid interruption of an ongoing event, as it may provoke a violent reaction. General nonpharmacologic measures already mentioned help in reducing the frequency of these events.

Pharmacotherapy can be considered for cases with frequent spells and bothersome complaints. Both BZDs, such as diazepam[115] and clonazepam,[102] and non-BZDs, such as imipramine[116] and paroxetine,[112] have been reported to be effective in alleviating complaints. Use of L-5-hydroxytryptophan has also been reported to be effective in treating sleep terrors. The effect of this treatment may last for up to 6 months.[117]

SUMMARY

Disorders of arousal, commonly seen in children and adults, occur during slow-wave sleep, usually during the first third of the night. The activities performed during an event may vary in their complexity, with individuals having an impaired recall of the events on awakening. Several factors may predispose an individual to these disorders. Previous family history also significantly increases the likelihood of developing a disorder of arousal. Most of these individuals have no underlying psychiatric condition. It is important to differentiate these disorders from RBD, NFLE, and other neuropsychiatric disorders capable of mimicking them. Video PSG with extensive EEG monitoring is the investigation of choice to confirm the diagnosis and rule out other sleep disorders. Further research is needed to develop a standard protocol for conducting optimal sleep studies in patients with suspected disorders of arousal. The role of sleep deprivation and auditory stimuli needs to be explored in this regard. Treatment involves prevention of triggers, creation of a safe sleep environment, and use of pharmacotherapy in resistant cases.

ACKNOWLEDGMENTS

The authors wish to acknowledge Dr Christian Guilleminault and Dr Chad Rouff, (Stanford Center for Sleep Sciences and Medicine) for providing the image of a polysomnogram and details of the patient with parasomnia.

REFERENCES

1. Mahowald MW, Schenck CH. Status dissociatus–a perspective on states of being. Sleep 1991;14(1): 69–79.
2. Mahowald MW, Bornemann MA, Kryger MH, et al. Non-REM arousal parasomnias. Chapter 94. In: Principles and practice of sleep medicine. 5th edition. Philadelphia: W.B. Saunders; 2011. p. 1075–82.
3. Mahowald MW, Schenck CH. Dissociated states of wakefulness and sleep. Neurology 1992;42(7 Suppl 6):44–51 [discussion: 52].
4. Mahowald MW, Schenck CH. Evolving concepts of human state dissociation. Arch Ital Biol 2001; 139(3):269–300.
5. American Academy of Sleep Medicine. International classification of sleep disorders. 3rd edition. Darien (IL): American Academy of Sleep Medicine; 2014.
6. Liu X, Ma Y, Wang Y, et al. Brief report: an epidemiologic survey of the prevalence of sleep disorders among children 2 to 12 years old in Beijing, China. Pediatrics 2005;115(Suppl 1):266–8.
7. Klackenberg G. Somnambulism in childhood–prevalence, course and behavioral correlations. A prospective longitudinal study (6-16 years). Acta Paediatr Scand 1982;71(3):495–9.
8. Petit D, Touchette E, Tremblay RE, et al. Dyssomnias and parasomnias in early childhood. Pediatrics 2007;119(5):e1016–25.
9. Ohayon MM, Guilleminault C, Priest RG. Night terrors, sleepwalking, and confusional arousals in the general population: their frequency and relationship to other sleep and mental disorders. J Clin Psychiatry 1999;60(4):268–76 [quiz: 277].
10. Hublin C, Kaprio J, Partinen M, et al. Prevalence and genetics of sleepwalking: a population-based twin study. Neurology 1997;48(1):177–81.
11. Ohayon MM, Mahowald MW, Dauvilliers Y, et al. Prevalence and comorbidity of nocturnal wandering in the U.S. adult general population. Neurology 2012;78(20):1583–9.
12. Barclay NL, Gregory AM. Quantitative genetic research on sleep: a review of normal sleep, sleep disturbances and associated emotional, behavioural, and health-related difficulties. Sleep Med Rev 2013;17(1):29–40.
13. Licis AK, Desruisseau DM, Yamada KA, et al. Novel genetic findings in an extended family pedigree with sleepwalking. Neurology 2011;76(1):49–52.
14. Nobili L, Ferrara M, Moroni F, et al. Dissociated wake-like and sleep-like electro-cortical activity during sleep. Neuroimage 2011;58(2):612–9.
15. Mahowald MW, Schenck CH. Insights from studying human sleep disorders. Nature 2005; 437(7063):1279–85.
16. Terzaghi M, Sartori I, Tassi L, et al. Evidence of dissociated arousal states during NREM parasomnia from an intracerebral neurophysiological study. Sleep 2009;32(3):409–12.
17. Bassetti C, Vella S, Donati F, et al. SPECT during sleepwalking. Lancet 2000;356(9228):484–5.
18. Nir Y, Staba RJ, Andrillon T, et al. Regional slow waves and spindles in human sleep. Neuron 2011;70(1):153–69.
19. Guilleminault C, Lee JH, Chan A, et al. Non-REM-sleep instability in recurrent sleepwalking in pre-pubertal children. Sleep Med 2005;6(6):515–21.
20. Parrino L, Halasz P, Tassinari CA, et al. CAP, epilepsy and motor events during sleep: the unifying role of arousal. Sleep Med Rev 2006;10(4):267–85.
21. Zadra A, Desautels A, Petit D, et al. Somnambulism: clinical aspects and pathophysiological hypotheses. Lancet Neurol 2013;12(3):285–94.
22. Pilon M, Montplaisir J, Zadra A. Precipitating factors of somnambulism: impact of sleep deprivation and forced arousals. Neurology 2008;70(24): 2284–90.
23. Espa F, Ondze B, Deglise P, et al. Sleep architecture, slow wave activity, and sleep spindles in adult patients with sleepwalking and sleep terrors. Clin Neurophysiol 2000;111(5):929–39.
24. Guilleminault C, Palombini L, Pelayo R, et al. Sleepwalking and sleep terrors in prepubertal children: what triggers them? Pediatrics 2003;111(1):e17–25.
25. Soldatos CR, Vela-Bueno A, Bixler EO, et al. Sleepwalking and night terrors in adulthood clinical EEG findings. Clin Electroencephalogr 1980;11(3):136–9.
26. Kales A, Soldatos CR, Caldwell AB, et al. Somnambulism. Clinical characteristics and personality patterns. Arch Gen Psychiatry 1980;37(12):1406–10.
27. Zadra A, Pilon M. NREM parasomnias. Handb Clin Neurol 2011;99:851–68.
28. Schenck CH, Mahowald MW. On the reported association of psychopathology with sleep terrors in adults. Sleep 2000;23(4):448–9.
29. Schenck CH, Milner DM, Hurwitz TD, et al. A polysomnographic and clinical report on sleep-related injury in 100 adult patients. Am J Psychiatry 1989;146(9):1166–73.
30. Pressman MR. Factors that predispose, prime and precipitate NREM parasomnias in adults: clinical and forensic implications. Sleep Med Rev 2007; 11(1):5–30 [discussion 31–3].
31. Pilon M, Desautels A, Montplaisir J, et al. Auditory arousal responses and thresholds during REM and NREM sleep of sleepwalkers and controls. Sleep Med 2012;13(5):490–5.
32. Perrault R, Carrier J, Desautels A, et al. Slow wave activity and slow oscillations in sleepwalkers and controls: effects of 38 h of sleep deprivation. J Sleep Res 2013;22(4):430–3.
33. Joncas S, Zadra A, Paquet J, et al. The value of sleep deprivation as a diagnostic tool in adult sleepwalkers. Neurology 2002;58(6):936–40.

34. Pilon M, Zadra A, Joncas S, et al. Hypersynchronous delta waves and somnambulism: brain topography and effect of sleep deprivation. Sleep 2006; 29(1):77–84.
35. Zadra A, Pilon M, Montplaisir J. Polysomnographic diagnosis of sleepwalking: effects of sleep deprivation. Ann Neurol 2008;63(4):513–9.
36. Yang W, Dollear M, Muthukrishnan SR. One rare side effect of zolpidem–sleepwalking: a case report. Arch Phys Med Rehabil 2005;86(6):1265–6.
37. Harazin J, Berigan TR. Zolpidem tartrate and somnambulism. Mil Med 1999;164(9):669–70.
38. Charney DS, Kales A, Soldatos CR, et al. Somnambulistic-like episodes secondary to combined lithium-neuroleptic treatment. Br J Psychiatry 1979; 135:418–24.
39. Menkes DB. Triazolam-induced nocturnal bingeing with amnesia. Aust N Z J Psychiatry 1992;26(2):320–1.
40. Kawashima T, Yamada S. Paroxetine-induced somnambulism. J Clin Psychiatry 2003;64(4):483.
41. Larsen CH, Dooley J, Gordon K. Fever-associated confusional arousal. Eur J Pediatr 2004;163(11): 696–7.
42. Snyder S. Unusual case of sleep terror in a pregnant patient. Am J Psychiatry 1986;143(3):391.
43. Berlin RM. Sleepwalking disorder during pregnancy: a case report. Sleep 1988;11(3):298–300.
44. Pressman MR, Mahowald MW, Schenck CH, et al. Alcohol, sleepwalking and violence: lack of reliable scientific evidence. Brain 2013;136(Pt 2):e229.
45. Lopez R, Jaussent I, Scholz S, et al. Functional impairment in adult sleepwalkers: a case-control study. Sleep 2013;36(3):345–51.
46. Pressman MR. Common misconceptions about sleepwalking and other parasomnias. Sleep Med Clin 2011;6(4):xiii–xvii.
47. Pressman MR. Disorders of arousal from sleep and violent behavior: the role of physical contact and proximity. Sleep 2007;30(8):1039–47.
48. Fisher C, Kahn E, Edwards A, et al. A psychophysiological study of nightmares and night terrors. I. Physiological aspects of the stage 4 night terror. J Nerv Ment Dis 1973;157(2):75–98.
49. Howell MJ, Schenck CH, Crow SJ. A review of nighttime eating disorders. Sleep Med Rev 2009; 13(1):23–34.
50. Brion A, Flamand M, Oudiette D, et al. Sleep-related eating disorder versus sleepwalking: a controlled study. Sleep Med 2012;13(8):1094–101.
51. Santin J, Mery V, Elso MJ, et al. Sleep-related eating disorder: a descriptive study in Chilean patients. Sleep Med 2014;15(2):163–7.
52. Schenck CH, Hurwitz TD, Bundlie SR, et al. Sleep-related eating disorders: polysomnographic correlates of a heterogeneous syndrome distinct from daytime eating disorders. Sleep 1991;14(5): 419–31.
53. Paquet V, Strul J, Servais L, et al. Sleep-related eating disorder induced by olanzapine. J Clin Psychiatry 2002;63(7):597.
54. Lu ML, Shen WW. Sleep-related eating disorder induced by risperidone. J Clin Psychiatry 2004; 65(2):273–4.
55. Hoque R, Chesson AL Jr. Zolpidem-induced sleepwalking, sleep related eating disorder, and sleep-driving: fluorine-18-flourodeoxyglucose positron emission tomography analysis, and a literature review of other unexpected clinical effects of zolpidem. J Clin Sleep Med 2009;5(5):471–6.
56. Nzwalo H, Ferreira L, Peralta R, et al. Sleep-related eating disorder secondary to zolpidem. BMJ Case Rep 2013;2013.
57. Schenck CH, Mahowald MW. Review of nocturnal sleep-related eating disorders. Int J Eat Disord 1994;15(4):343–56.
58. Vinai P, Ferri R, Ferini-Strambi L, et al. Defining the borders between sleep-related eating disorder and night eating syndrome. Sleep Med 2012;13(6):686–90.
59. Winkelman JW. Clinical and polysomnographic features of sleep-related eating disorder. J Clin Psychiatry 1998;59(1):14–9.
60. Provini F, Albani F, Vetrugno R, et al. A pilot double-blind placebo-controlled trial of low-dose pramipexole in sleep-related eating disorder. Eur J Neurol 2005;12(6):432–6.
61. Winkelman JW. Efficacy and tolerability of open-label topiramate in the treatment of sleep-related eating disorder: a retrospective case series. J Clin Psychiatry 2006;67(11):1729–34.
62. Winkelman JW. A randomized, double-blind, placebo-controlled, parallel group study to determine the efficacy and safety of topiramate in the treatment of sleep-related eating disorder. Bethesda (MD): National Library of Medicine (US); 2000–2014 [Internet]. Available at: Clinicaltrials.gov.
63. Buchanan PR. Sleep sex. Sleep Med Clin 2011; 6(4):417–28.
64. Shapiro CM, Trajanovic NN, Fedoroff JP. Sexsomnia–a new parasomnia? Can J Psychiatry 2003; 48(5):311–7.
65. Guilleminault C, Moscovitch A, Yuen K, et al. Atypical sexual behavior during sleep. Psychosom Med 2002;64(2):328–36.
66. Schenck CH, Arnulf I, Mahowald MW. Sleep and sex: what can go wrong? A review of the literature on sleep related disorders and abnormal sexual behaviors and experiences. Sleep 2007;30(6):683–702.
67. Schenck CH, Hurwitz TD. Other Parasomnias in Adults: Sexsomnia, Sleep-Related Dissociative Disorder, Catathrenia, Sleep-Related Hallucinations, and Sleep Talking. In: Barkoukis TJ, Matheson JK, Ferber R, et al, editors. Therapy in Sleep Medicine. First edition. Philadelphia, PA: Elsevier Health Sciences; 2012. p. 573–82.

68. Cicolin A, Tribolo A, Giordano A, et al. Sexual behaviors during sleep associated with polysomnographically confirmed parasomnia overlap disorder. Sleep Med 2011;12(5):523–8.
69. Nobili L. Can homemade video recording become more than a screening tool? Sleep 2009;32(12): 1544–5.
70. APA. Diagnostic and statistical manual of mental disorders. 5th edition. Arlingtion (VA): American Psychiatric Publishing; 2013.
71. Kushida CA, Littner MR, Morgenthaler T, et al. Practice parameters for the indications for polysomnography and related procedures: an update for 2005. Sleep 2005;28(4):499–521.
72. Tinuper P, Provini F, Bisulli F, et al. Movement disorders in sleep: guidelines for differentiating epileptic from non-epileptic motor phenomena arising from sleep. Sleep Med Rev 2007;11(4):255–67.
73. Tinuper P, Cerullo A, Cirignotta F, et al. Nocturnal paroxysmal dystonia with short-lasting attacks: three cases with evidence for an epileptic frontal lobe origin of seizures. Epilepsia 1990;31(5): 549–56.
74. Blatt I, Peled R, Gadoth N, et al. The value of sleep recording in evaluating somnambulism in young adults. Electroencephalogr Clin Neurophysiol 1991;78(6):407–12.
75. Gaudreau H, Joncas S, Zadra A, et al. Dynamics of slow-wave activity during the NREM sleep of sleepwalkers and control subjects. Sleep 2000;23(6): 755–60.
76. Guilleminault C. Hypersynchronous slow delta, cyclic alternating pattern and sleepwalking. Sleep 2006;29(1):14–5.
77. Halasz P, Kelemen A, Szucs A. Physiopathogenetic interrelationship between nocturnal frontal lobe epilepsy and NREM arousal parasomnias. Epilepsy Res Treat 2012;2012:312693.
78. Halasz P, Ujszaszi J, Gadoros J. Are microarousals preceded by electroencephalographic slow wave synchronization precursors of confusional awakenings? Sleep 1985;8(3):231–8.
79. Jaar O, Pilon M, Carrier J, et al. Analysis of slow-wave activity and slow-wave oscillations prior to somnambulism. Sleep 2010;33(11):1511–6.
80. Schenck CH, Bundlie SR, Ettinger MG, et al. Chronic behavioral disorders of human REM sleep: a new category of parasomnia. Sleep 1986;9(2):293–308.
81. Schenck CH, Mahowald MW. REM sleep behavior disorder: clinical, developmental, and neuroscience perspectives 16 years after its formal identification in SLEEP. Sleep 2002;25(2):120–38.
82. Schenck CH, Garcia-Rill E, Skinner RD, et al. A case of REM sleep behavior disorder with autopsy-confirmed Alzheimer's disease: postmortem brain stem histochemical analyses. Biol Psychiatry 1996;40(5):422–5.
83. Boeve BF, Silber MH, Ferman TJ, et al. Association of REM sleep behavior disorder and neurodegenerative disease may reflect an underlying synucleinopathy. Mov Disord 2001;16(4):622–30.
84. Mahowald MW, Schenck CH, Kryger MH, et al. REM sleep parasomnias. Chapter 95. In: Principles and practice of sleep medicine. 5th edition. Philadelphia: W.B. Saunders; 2011. p. 1083–97.
85. Schenck CH, Boyd JL, Mahowald MW. A parasomnia overlap disorder involving sleepwalking, sleep terrors, and REM sleep behavior disorder in 33 polysomnographically confirmed cases. Sleep 1997;20(11): 972–81.
86. Nobili L, Proserpio P, Combi R, et al. Nocturnal frontal lobe epilepsy. Curr Neurol Neurosci Rep 2014;14(2):424.
87. Derry CP, Davey M, Johns M, et al. Distinguishing sleep disorders from seizures: diagnosing bumps in the night. Arch Neurol 2006;63(5):705–9.
88. Zaiwalla Z. Parasomnias. Clin Med 2005;5(2):109–12.
89. Zucconi M, Ferini-Strambi L. NREM parasomnias: arousal disorders and differentiation from nocturnal frontal lobe epilepsy. Clin Neurophysiol 2000; 111(Suppl 2):S129–35.
90. Derry CP, Harvey AS, Walker MC, et al. NREM arousal parasomnias and their distinction from nocturnal frontal lobe epilepsy: a video EEG analysis. Sleep 2009;32(12):1637–44.
91. Vignatelli L, Bisulli F, Provini F, et al. Interobserver reliability of video recording in the diagnosis of nocturnal frontal lobe seizures. Epilepsia 2007;48(8):1506–11.
92. Terzaghi M, Sartori I, Mai R, et al. Sleep-related minor motor events in nocturnal frontal lobe epilepsy. Epilepsia 2007;48(2):335–41.
93. Bisulli F, Vignatelli L, Naldi I, et al. Diagnostic accuracy of a structured interview for nocturnal frontal lobe epilepsy (SINFLE): a proposal for developing diagnostic criteria. Sleep Med 2012;13(1):81–7.
94. Provini F, Plazzi G, Tinuper P, et al. Nocturnal frontal lobe epilepsy. A clinical and polygraphic overview of 100 consecutive cases. Brain 1999;122(Pt 6): 1017–31.
95. Manni R, Terzaghi M, Repetto A. The FLEP scale in diagnosing nocturnal frontal lobe epilepsy, NREM and REM parasomnias: data from a tertiary sleep and epilepsy unit. Epilepsia 2008;49(9):1581–5.
96. Craske MG, Tsao JC. Assessment and treatment of nocturnal panic attacks. Sleep Med Rev 2005;9(3): 173–84.
97. Isik U, D'Cruz O. Cluster headaches simulating parasomnias. Pediatr Neurol 2002;27(3):227–9.
98. Glaze DG, Frost JD Jr, Jankovic J. Sleep in Gilles de la Tourette's syndrome: disorder of arousal. Neurology 1983;33(5):586–92.
99. Barabas G, Matthews WS, Ferrari M. Disorders of arousal in Gilles de la Tourette's syndrome. Neurology 1984;34(6):815–7.

100. Casez O, Dananchet Y, Besson G. Migraine and somnambulism. Neurology 2005;65(8):1334–5.
101. Johnson H, Wiggs L, Stores G, et al. Psychological disturbance and sleep disorders in children with neurofibromatosis type 1. Dev Med Child Neurol 2005;47(4):237–42.
102. Schenck CH, Mahowald MW. Therapeutics for parasomnias in adults. Sleep Med Clin 2010;5(4): 689–700.
103. Attarian H. Treatment options for parasomnias. Neurol Clin 2010;28(4):1089–106.
104. Frank NC, Spirito A, Stark L, et al. The use of scheduled awakenings to eliminate childhood sleepwalking. J Pediatr Psychol 1997;22(3): 345–53.
105. Mahowald MW, Schenck CH. Non-rapid eye movement sleep parasomnias. Neurol Clin 2005;23(4): 1077–106, vii.
106. Reid WH, Ahmed I, Levie CA. Treatment of sleepwalking: a controlled study. Am J Psychother 1981;35(1):27–37.
107. Hauri PJ, Silber MH, Boeve BF. The treatment of parasomnias with hypnosis: a 5-year follow-up study. J Clin Sleep Med 2007;3(4):369–73.
108. Harris M, Grunstein RR. Treatments for somnambulism in adults: assessing the evidence. Sleep Med Rev 2009;13(4):295–7.
109. Schenck CH, Mahowald MW. Long-term, nightly benzodiazepine treatment of injurious parasomnias and other disorders of disrupted nocturnal sleep in 170 adults. Am J Med 1996;100(3):333–7.
110. Remulla A, Guilleminault C. Somnambulism (sleepwalking). Expert Opin Pharmacother 2004;5(10): 2069–74.
111. Berlin RM, Qayyum U. Sleepwalking: diagnosis and treatment through the life cycle. Psychosomatics 1986;27(11):755–60.
112. Lillywhite AR, Wilson SJ, Nutt DJ. Successful treatment of night terrors and somnambulism with paroxetine. Br J Psychiatry 1994;164(4):551–4.
113. Jan JE, Freeman RD, Wasdell MB, et al. A child with severe night terrors and sleep-walking responds to melatonin therapy. Dev Med Child Neurol 2004;46(11):789.
114. Mason TB 2nd, Pack AI. Pediatric parasomnias. Sleep 2007;30(2):141–51.
115. Allen RM. Attenuation of drug-induced anxiety dreams and pavor nocturnus by benzodiazepines. J Clin Psychiatry 1983;44(3):106–8.
116. Burstein A. Treatment of night terrors with imipramine. J Clin Psychiatry 1983;44(2):82.
117. Bruni O, Ferri R, Miano S, et al. L-5-Hydroxytryptophan treatment of sleep terrors in children. Eur J Pediatr 2004;163(7):402–7.

Nightmares and Dream-Enactment Behaviors

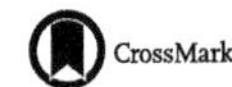

Mia Zaharna, MD, MPH

KEYWORDS

• Nightmares • Parasomnias • REM behavior disorder • Dreaming • Sleepwalking • REM sleep

KEY POINTS

- Parasomnias are undesirable motor, verbal, or experiential phenomena occurring in sleep and may be primary rapid eye movement (REM) or non-REM parasomnias or secondary parasomnias.
- Nightmare disorder and REM behavior disorder (RBD) are 2 types of primary parasomnias.
- RBD occurs when a person begins to physically act out a dream during the REM stage of sleep. These dreams tend to be unpleasant, action filled, or violent and often result in self-injury or injury to one's bed partner.
- RBD is often associated with the development of neurodegenerative disorders, such as Parkinson disease, multiple system atrophy, Lewy body dementia, and others.
- Nightmares are disturbing mental experiences that tend to occur during REM sleep. Episodes are often vivid and terrifying, result in awakening from sleep, and are often easily recalled.

INTRODUCTION

Normal behaviors in sleep are shown in **Box 1**. Parasomnias are disorders characterized by undesirable motor, verbal, or experiential phenomena occurring in association with sleep, specific stages of sleep, or sleep-awake transition phases.[1] Parasomnias are divided into 2 major categories: primary parasomnias (**Box 2**), which are disorders of sleep states, and secondary parasomnias (**Box 3**), which are caused by disorders of other organ systems that may manifest during sleep. Primary parasomnias are further subclassified as non–rapid eye movement (NREM) or rapid eye movement (REM) parasomnias. Associated abnormal movements, behaviors, emotions, perceptions, and dreams may occur. Actions associated with parasomnias are not consciously controlled and can result in physical injuries. Parasomnias can also result in adverse health effects, psychological disturbances, and disrupted sleep.

This article focuses on nightmares and dream-enactment behaviors, which are 2 categories of REM-related parasomnias.

NIGHTMARES AND DREAM-ENACTMENT BEHAVIORS

Introduction

Dreams occur during all stages of sleep. Dreaming is a sleep-related cognitive activity characterized by multisensory imagery, emotional arousal, and apparent speech and motor activity.[2] Although some researchers think dreams have no function, others suggest dreams are a continuation of daytime conscious thought processing.[3] Dreaming may be important for learning, memory processing, and adaptation to emotional and physical stress.[4]

Nightmares are disturbing mental experiences that tend to occur during REM sleep. Episodes are often vivid and terrifying and result in awakening from sleep. The dreamer is often able to recall details of the nightmare, and themes often involve physical danger and emotional distress. Difficulty returning to sleep after a nightmare is common.

Nightmares may be unassociated with any underlying psychopathology. However, mental health issues, including posttraumatic stress disorder (PTSD), substance abuse, stress, anxiety,

The author has nothing to disclose.
Kaiser San Jose Division of Sleep Medicine, The Permanente Medical Group, Inc, 275 Hospital Parkway, Suite #425, San Jose, CA 95119, USA
E-mail address: mia.zaharna@gmail.com

Sleep Med Clin 9 (2014) 553–560
http://dx.doi.org/10.1016/j.jsmc.2014.08.004
1556-407X/14/$ – see front matter

Box 1
Normal behaviors in sleep

Sleep starts: motor or sensory

Exploding head syndrome

Explosive tinnitus

Sleep paralysis

Hypnogogic/hypnopompic hallucinations

borderline personality disorder, and schizophrenia spectrum disorders, have been associated with nightmares.[5] PTSD-associated nightmares have been the most studied. In fact, nightmares are part of the diagnostic criteria symptom cluster of intrusive/reexperiencing of the traumatic event. Eighty percent of patients with PTSD report PTSD-associated nightmares.[6] Nightmares have also been associated with drug use (norepinephrine, serotonin, and dopamine acting drugs) and withdrawal from drugs (REM-suppressing, γ-aminobutyric acid [GABA], and acetylcholine-affecting drugs).[7,8]

Definition

Nightmare disorder

Nightmare disorder develops when a person frequently has recurrent nightmares that produce awakenings from sleep (**Box 4**). These nightmares may keep the person from returning to sleep, and they often occur in the latter half of the sleep period when REM sleep stages are longer.

Rapid-eye-movement behavior disorder

REM behavior disorder (RBD) occurs when a person begins to physically act out a dream during the REM stage of sleep (**Box 5**). These dreams tend to be unpleasant, action filled, or violent. Often the

Box 2
Primary parasomnias

NREM

- Confusional arousals
- Sleepwalking
- Sleep terrors

REM

- REM behavior disorder
- Nightmares
- REM-related painful erections

Abbreviations: NREM, non–rapid eye movement; REM, rapid eye movement.

Box 3
Secondary parasomnias

Central nervous system

- Seizures
- Headaches
- Exploding head syndrome
- Tinnitus

Cardiopulmonary parasomnias

- Arrhythmias
- Nocturnal angina pectoris
- Nocturnal asthma
- Respiratory dyskinesias
- Sleep hiccups
- Choking
- Coughing

Gastrointestinal parasomnias

- Gastroesophageal reflux disease
- Diffuse esophageal spasm
- Abnormal swallowing

Miscellaneous

- Nocturnal muscle cramps
- Nocturnal pruritus
- Night sweats

Benign nocturnal hemiplegia of childhood

Box 4
Nightmare disorder

1. Recurrent episodes of awakenings from sleep with recall of intensely disturbing dream mentations, usually involving fear or anxiety but also anger, sadness, disgust, and other dysphoric emotions
2. Full alertness on awakening, with little confusion or disorientation; immediate and clear recall of sleep mentation
3. Presence of at least one of the following associated features:
   a. Delayed return to sleep after the episodes
   b. Occurrence of episodes in the latter half of the habitual sleep period

From American Academy of Sleep Medicine. International classification of sleep disorders. In: Sateia M, editor. Diagnostic and coding manual. 3rd edition. Darien (IL): American Academy of Sleep Medicine; 2014; with permission.

Box 5
REM behavior disorder

1. Presence of REM sleep without atonia: the electromyogram (EMG) finding of excessive amounts of sustained or intermittent elevation of submental EMG tone or excessive phasic submental or (upper or lower) limb EMG twitching
2. At least one of the following is present:
   a. Sleep-related injurious, potentially injurious, or disruptive behaviors by history
   b. Abnormal REM sleep behaviors documented during polysomnographic monitoring
   c. Awakening short of breath
3. Absence of electroencephalogram (EEG) epileptiform activity during REM sleep unless RBD can be clearly distinguished from concurrent REM sleep-related seizure disorder
4. The sleep disturbance not better explained by another sleep disorder, medical or neurologic disorder, mental disorder, medication use, or substance use disorder

From American Academy of Sleep Medicine. International classification of sleep disorders. In: Sateia M, editor. Diagnostic and coding manual. 3rd edition. Darien (IL): American Academy of Sleep Medicine; 2014; with permission.

dreamer is being confronted, attacked, or chased by a person or animal. On waking from an episode, the sleeper typically becomes rapidly alert and can describe a dream with a coherent story that corresponds with the unusual actions. This disorder is a male-predominant disorder that usually emerges after 50 years of age, although any age group can be affected. Major predisposing factors for RBD include sex, age, and an underlying neurologic disorder, particularly parkinsonism, dementia, narcolepsy, and stroke. An increasingly recognized precipitating factor is medicine use, particularly of selective serotonin reuptake inhibitors, mirtazapine, and other antidepressant agents with the exception of bupropion. In children and adolescents, predisposing factors for RBD include narcolepsy, the use of psychotropic medications, brainstem tumors, parkinsonism, Tourette syndrome, and autism.

Symptom criteria

Nightmare disorder

- Repeated awakenings from sleep caused by frightening dreams
- Generally occur during the second half of the sleep period
- May result in anxiety, depression, sleep avoidance and sleep deprivation, insomnia, daytime sleepiness, fatigue, or other psychological dysfunction[9–11]

Rapid-eye-movement behavior disorder

- Dream-enacting behaviors, often violent
- Usually nondirected behaviors and may include punching, kicking, leaping from bed while still asleep
- May wake spontaneously during the attack
- Often vividly remembers the dream
- Often results in self-injury or injury to the bed partner

CLINICAL FINDINGS

Physical Examination

Parasomnias are sometimes misdiagnosed as psychiatric disorders. Parasomnias may be primary sleep disorders or secondary to underlying medical or psychiatric disorders, so evaluation by a sleep medicine expert is recommended.

Although the diagnosis of parasomnias, including RBD and nightmare disorder, is often elucidated through a good clinical history and patient interview, care must be taken to rule out underlying medical and neurologic disorders through a physical examination and targeted medical history.

The physical examination should contain a complete neurologic examination, as RBD has been associated with the emergence of neurodegenerative disorders, such as Parkinson disease, multiple system atrophy (MSA), Lewy body dementia, and others. The symptoms of these diseases are listed in **Box 6**. One study showed 38% of 50-year-old men with RBD and no neurologic signs went on to develop parkinsonism.[12] Ninety percent of patients with MSA have RBD. Although rare, seizure disorders may also present as nightmares or associated with dream-enactment behaviors.

Rating Scales

Specific rating scales are generally not used to distinguish parasomnias. Self-reported retrospective questionnaires and prospective logs are the most commonly used methods to assess nightmares.[5] When suspicion for PTSD is present in association with nightmares, the Clinician Administered PTSD Scale (CAPS) may be used. CAPS is the gold standard diagnostic interview for PTSD and assesses the frequency and intensity of 17 symptoms, including nightmares.[13] For further review of related psychiatric conditions, the Symptom Questionnaire (SQ) may be used. The SQ is a brief yes/no questionnaire that includes items on state scales of depression, anxiety, anger-hostility, and

Box 6
Symptoms of neurodegenerative disorders in the differential diagnosis for RBD

Parkinson disease

- Resting tremor
- Rigidity
- Bradykinesia
- Postural instability
- Laryngeal dysfunction and dysphagia
- Autonomic instability

Multiple systems atrophy

- Autonomic and/or urinary dysfunction
- Severe orthostatic hypotension-lightheadedness, dizziness, dimming of vision, weakness, fatigue, yawning, slurred speech, syncope
- Parkinsonism-tremor, rigidity, bradykinesia, ataxia
- Cerebellar dysfunction-gait and limb ataxia, tremor, myoclonus

Lewy body dementia

- Visual hallucinations
- Parkinsonian motor features
- Cognitive dysfunction

somatic symptoms.[14] Rating scales are generally not used in the evaluation of RBD.

Diagnostic Modalities

No specific laboratory studies or imaging studies are necessary in the diagnosis of parasomnias. However, laboratory work or imaging may be helpful in uncovering underlying medical disorders that may be the cause of the parasomnia. Periodic limb movements in sleep (PLMS) are very common in patients with RBD. In cases of restless legs syndrome and/or PLMS, a serum ferritin level, complete blood count, and serum iron levels may be ordered to determine the presence of anemia and low iron stores.

Polysomnography with video recording is essential in the diagnosis of RBD. Intermittent loss of REM atonia, excessive amount of sustained electromyogram (EMG) activity, or excessive phasic muscle twitch activity of the submental or limb EMG during REM sleep is present. Although an increased heart rate is a feature of normal REM sleep, autonomic nervous system activation is uncommon during REM sleep in RBD.

Although polysomnography is not required in the diagnosis of nightmare disorder, it may be used to exclude the presence of other parasomnias or a sleep-related breathing disorder.

PATHOLOGY

The precise pathophysiology of parasomnias is unknown.

The cause of RBD is thought to be associated with sleep-regulating nuclei known as the pontine tegmentum. Neurochemical systems, such as the noradrenergic, cholinergic, and serotoninergic systems, may also be involved.[15,16] Various pontine nuclei are known to influence the REM and non-REM sleep circuits, including the locus coeruleus, pedunculopontine nucleus, and laterodorsal tegmental nucleus.[17] In addition, forebrain cortical and subcortical structures and the substantia nigra, thalamus, hypothalamus, basal forebrain, and frontal cortex are also involved; but their precise role is unknown.

RBD has been experimentally produced in the laboratory in cats by bilateral pontine tegmental lesions, which are associated with the absence of REM atony. In humans, most patients with RBD do not have an identifiable neurologic disorder or structural neuropathology. Muscle atony in REM sleep in humans may be caused by functional dysregulation by depression of brainstem structures responsible for inhibiting phasic activity.

The cause of nightmare disorder is unknown. Nightmares have been associated with pharmacologic agents affecting the neurotransmitters norepinephrine, serotonin, and dopamine. Withdrawal from REM-suppressing agents and agents affecting the GABA, acetylcholine, and histamine neurotransmitter systems have also been associated with nightmares.

DIAGNOSTIC DILEMMAS

Differential Diagnosis

Nightmare disorder and RBD are often misdiagnosed as psychiatric disorders. The differential diagnosis includes various psychiatric disorders as well as underlying medical and neurologic disorders (**Boxes 7** and **8**). Various primary sleep disorders can also be contributors to symptoms of nightmares and dream-enactment behaviors.

Process of Elimination

Distinguishing between various parasomnias and between parasomnias and seizure disorders can be done by a detailed clinical history and, when necessary, an overnight polysomnogram. A seizure montage on electroencephalogram (EEG) may be

Box 7
Differential diagnosis for nightmare disorder

- Primary sleep disorders
  - Sleep terrors
  - RBD
  - Narcolepsy, often nightmares are reported at sleep onset
- Medical and neurologic disorders
  - Seizure disorder
- Psychiatric disorders
  - PTSD
  - Nocturnal panic attacks
  - Sleep-related dissociative disorders
  - Substance abuse disorders

From American Academy of Sleep Medicine. International classification of sleep disorders. In: Sateia M, editor. Diagnostic and coding manual. 3rd edition. Darien (IL): American Academy of Sleep Medicine; 2014; with permission.

necessary to determine the presence of epileptiform activity. Some key distinguishing features, such as the presence or absence of memory for the event, associated symptoms, sleep stage of event occurrence, and polysomnographic features, can be used to assist in the diagnosis (**Table 1**).

TREATMENT

The treatment of parasomnias, nightmares, and dream-enactment behaviors may be unnecessary, as such episodes often occur in healthy people. However, if the parasomnia is disturbing to patients or bed partners or if it results in dangerous behaviors, treatment may be warranted. Parasomnias that develop in childhood often improve with age.

A comprehensive treatment plan for parasomnias may include improvement in sleep hygiene, cognitive behavioral therapy (CBT) to overcome fear and anxiety related to the parasomnia, and medications. The use of alcohol and drugs and sleep deprivation may worsen parasomnias, so avoidance of these behaviors should be encouraged. Hypnotic medications may improve sleep and lessen the presence of parasomnias.

Nightmare disorder may be treated with medications and/or behavioral therapies. Most of the treatment recommendations focus on PTSD-associated nightmares (**Box 9**). Prazosin, an alpha-1 adrenergic receptor antagonist, is recommended for the treatment of PTSD-associated nightmares. However, patients should be monitored for orthostatic hypotension. Clonidine, an alpha-2 adrenergic receptor agonist, may also be considered for the treatment of PTSD associated nightmares. Clonidine may also result in orthostatic hypotension. Clonidine has not been as well studied as prazosin and, therefore, should be considered a secondary treatment option in PTSD-related nightmare disorder. Trazodone, low-dose atypical antipsychotics, topiramate, low-dose cortisol, fluvoxamine, triazolam, nitrazepam, phenelzine, gabapentin, cyproheptadine, and tricyclic antidepressants may all be considered for the treatment of PTSD-associated nightmares.

Box 8
Differential diagnosis for RBD

- Primary sleep disorders
  - Sleep terrors
  - Sleepwalking
  - Confusional arousals
  - Obstructive sleep apnea
  - PLMS
- Medical and neurologic disorders
  - Nocturnal seizure, frontal lobe epilepsy
  - Benign childhood epilepsy
  - Benign neonatal convulsions
  - Complex partial seizures
  - Confusional states and acute memory disorders
  - Dizziness, vertigo, and imbalance
  - Epilepsia partialis continua
  - Epilepsy, juvenile myoclonic
  - Epileptic and epileptiform encephalopathies
  - Frontal lobe epilepsy
- Psychiatric disorders
  - Psychogenic nonepileptic seizures
  - PTSD
  - Psychogenic dissociative disease
  - Malingering

From American Academy of Sleep Medicine. International classification of sleep disorders. In: Sateia M, editor. Diagnostic and coding manual. 3rd edition. Darien (IL): American Academy of Sleep Medicine; 2014; with permission.

Table 1
Key features for distinguishing abnormal behaviors in sleep

Night terrors	• Occurs in N3 sleep • No memory for episodes • Usually in first third of the night • Attempts to console may worsen the episode
Sleepwalking	• Occurs in N3 sleep • No memory for episodes • Usually eyes are open with a glassy stare
RBD	• Occurs in REM sleep • Dream-enactment behaviors • Loss of REM atonia on sleep study • Memory for dream content
Restless legs syndrome	• Symptoms of leg discomfort, worse at rest • Temporarily relieved by movement
Nightmare disorder	• Recurrent nightmares producing awakenings • Difficulty returning to sleep • Usually in second half of the night • Little confusion or disorientation involved
Sleep-related epilepsy	• May present in various forms from violent convulsions to little or no movement • May be associated with symptoms such as headache, injury, enuresis, tongue biting, or no symptoms at all • Abnormal EEG activity can confirm presence of seizures

Box 9
Treatment of PTSD-associated nightmares

Pharmacotherapy

- First line: prazosin
- Second line: clonidine
- Alternative options
  - Trazodone
  - Atypical antipsychotics: risperidone, aripiprazole, and olanzapine
  - Topiramate
  - Low-dose cortisol
  - Fluvoxamine
  - Triazolam and nitrazepam
  - Phenelzine
  - Gabapentin
  - Cyproheptadine
  - Tricyclic antidepressants

CBT

- First line: image rehearsal therapy
- Second line:
  - Systematic desensitization
  - Progressive deep muscle relaxation
- Alternative options
  - Lucid Dreaming Therapy
  - Exposure, relaxation, and rescripting therapy
  - Sleep dynamic therapy
  - Self-exposure therapy
  - Hypnosis
  - Eye movement desensitization and reprocessing
  - Testimony method

Nightmare disorder may be influenced by psychological factors, and psychotherapeutic approaches to treatment have been found effective. CBT has been shown to be effective in the treatment of PTSD-associated nightmares. CBT focuses on altering distorted thoughts, emotions, and behaviors through a structured approach. Specific types of CBT have been used to target symptoms of nightmares, including image rehearsal therapy, lucid dreaming therapy, sleep dynamic therapy, self-exposure therapy, and systematic desensitization. Image rehearsal therapy is the most highly recommended of these CBT techniques. It involves recall of the nightmare, writing it down, recomposition of the dream to a more positive one by changing some part of it, and rehearsal of the rewritten dream scenario. This method acts to change the original nightmare to a more positive dream when the nightmare should occur.

The treatment of RBD includes pharmacotherapy and injury prevention (**Box 10**). If pseudo-RBD is present, treatment of the underlying sleep pathology is first recommended.

The primary medications to be considered for the treatment of RBD are clonazepam and melatonin. Clonazepam is a long-acting benzodiazepine that has been shown to be effective in minimizing RBD behaviors. Its exact mechanism of action is

Box 10
Treatment of RBD

Pharmacotherapy

- First line: clonazepam
- Second line: melatonin
- Alternatives
  - Pramipexole
  - L-dopa
  - Paroxetine
  - Acetylcholinesterase inhibitors
  - Zopiclone
  - Temazepam, triazolam, alprazolam
  - Desipramine
  - Clozapine
  - Carbamazepine
  - Sodium oxybate

Injury Prevention

unknown. It has not been associated with a decrease in REM sleep or improvement of REM atonia.[18] The recommended dose is 0.25 mg to 2.0 mg 30 minutes before bedtime. The most common side effects included sedation, impotence, early morning motor incoordination, confusion, and memory dysfunction. Melatonin 3 to 12 mg at bedtime has been shown to be effective in the treatment of RBD. The data for the effectiveness of melatonin in the treatment of RBD are less strong than that of clonazepam, as few studies with a small number of patients have been done.[19–23] The side effects of melatonin include morning headache, morning sleepiness, and delusions/hallucinations. Pramipexole, L-dopa, and paroxetine may improve RBD but have also been shown to worsen dream-enactment behaviors.

SUMMARY

Parasomnias are undesirable emotional or physical events that accompany sleep. Parasomnias may be secondary to underlying medical disorders or sleep disorders, and a detailed clinical history and physical examination are necessary to appropriately diagnose the presence of a primary or secondary parasomnia. RBD and nightmare disorder are 2 types of parasomnias that generally occur during REM sleep. Although the treatment of parasomnias is not always necessary, it is often warranted because of the resulting adverse health effects, psychological disturbances, and disrupted sleep. Certain parasomnias like RBD often result in self-injury or injury to bed partners. Treatment is recommended in such cases, and precautionary measures to reduce potential for injury are important.

REFERENCES

1. Thorpy MJ, Glovinsky PB. Parasomnias. Psychiatr Clin North Am 1987;10(4):623–39.
2. Neilsen TN, Svob C, Kuiken D. Dream-enacting behaviors in a normal population. Sleep 2009; 32(12):1629–36.
3. Hobson JA. Dreaming as delirium: a mental status analysis of our nightly madness. Semin Neurol 1997;17:121–8.
4. Pagel JF. Nightmares and disorders of dreaming. Am Fam Physician 2000;61(7):2037–42.
5. Aurora NR, Zak RS, Auerbach SH, et al. Best practice guide for the treatment of nightmare disorder in adults. J Clin Sleep Med 2010;6(4):389–401.
6. Kilpatrick D, Resnick H, Freedy J, et al. Post-traumatic stress disorder field trial: evaluation of PTSD construct criteria A through E. In: Widiger T, Frances A, Pincus H, et al, editors. DSM-IV Sourcebook, vol. 4. Washington, DC: American Psychiatric Press; 1994. p. 803–38.
7. Pagel JF, Helfter P. Drug induced nightmares- an etiology based review. Hum Psychopharmacol 2003;18:59–67.
8. American Academy of Sleep Medicine. International classification of sleep disorders. In: Sateia M, editor. Diagnostic and coding manual. 2nd edition. Westchester (IL): American Academy of Sleep Medicine; 2005. p. 155–8.
9. DeViva JC, Zayfert C, Mellman TA. Factors associated with insomnia among civilians seeking treatment for PTSD: an exploratory study. Behav Sleep Med 2004;2:162–76.
10. Krakow B, Artar A, Warner TD, et al. Sleep disorder, depression, and suicidality in female sexual assault survivors. Crisis 2000;21:163–70.
11. Zayfert C, DeViva J. Residual insomnia following cognitive behavioral therapy for PTSD. J Trauma Stress 2004;17:69–73.
12. Simuni T, Sethi K. Nonmotor manifestations of Parkinson's disease. Ann Neurol 2008;64(Suppl 2): S65–80.
13. Blake DD, Weathers FW, Nagy LM, et al. The development of a clinician-administered PTSD scale. J Trauma Stress 1995;8:75–90.
14. Kellner RA. Symptom questionnaire. J Clin Psychiatry 1987;48:268–74.
15. Boeve BF, Silber MH, Saper CB, et al. Pathophysiology of REM sleep behaviour disorder and relevance to neurodegenerative disease. Brain 2007; 130:2770–88.

16. Hendricks JC, Morrison AR, Mann GL. Different behaviors during paradoxical sleep without atonia depend on pontine lesion site. Brain Res 1982; 239(1):81–105.
17. Rye DB. Contributions of the pedunculopontine region to normal and altered REM sleep. Sleep 1997;20(9):757–88.
18. Mahowald MW, Schenck CH, Bornemann MA. Pathophysiologic mechanisms in REM sleep behavior disorder. Curr Neurol Neurosci Rep 2007; 7:167–72.
19. Anderson KN, Shneerson JM. Drug treatment of REM sleep behavior disorder: the use of drug therapies other than clonazepam. J Clin Sleep Med 2009; 5:235–9.
20. Kunz D, Bes F. Melatonin effects in a patient with severe REM sleep behavior disorder: case report and theoretical considerations. Neuropsychobiology 1997;36:211–4.
21. Kunz D, Bes F. Melatonin as a therapy in REM sleep behavior disorder patients: an open-labeled pilot study on the possible influence of melatonin on REM-sleep regulation. Mov Disord 1999;14:507–11.
22. Takeuchi N, Uchimura N, Hashizume Y, et al. Melatonin therapy for REM sleep behavior disorder. Psychiatry Clin Neurosci 2001;55:267–9.
23. Boeve BF, Silber MH, Ferman TJ. Melatonin for treatment of REM sleep behavior disorder in neurologic disorders: results in 14 patients. Sleep Med 2003; 4:281–4.

Jet Lag and Shift Work

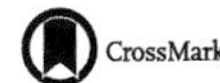

Robert E. Weir, MB BS, MRCOphth, MD[a], Chad C. Hagen, MD[b,*]

KEYWORDS

• Jet lag • Shift work disorder • Melatonin • Circadian rhythm • Sleep schedule • Phase shift

KEY POINTS

- Jet lag disorder and shift work disorder result from extrinsic work and travel obligations in conflict with the intrinsic circadian rhythm.
- Poor seasonal or ambient light can prolong the time to adapt to either transmeridian travel or shift work.
- Symptoms of extrinsic circadian disorders are similar to those of other sleep disorders; namely sleepiness, fatigue, poor or irritable moods, or cognitive inefficiency.
- Misalignment and the secondary effects are usually temporary and reversed over a period of days to weeks, given sufficient opportunity to recuperate and reentrain.

INTRODUCTION

The circadian rhythm orchestrates the rest/activity cycle with influences directly affecting cells throughout the brain and body. Although innate and coded within human DNA, this cycle usually does not run freely; it is modified by the circadian pacemaker interaction with circadian clock mechanisms. The pacemaker activity is a function of cells in the suprachiasmatic nucleus (SCN), within the hypothalamus. Cells throughout the brain and body have receptors modulating circadian molecular function and in turn affecting cellular activity and metabolism.[1] These rhythms can be regulated by zeitgebers, which are stimuli such as light, activity, or other sources of feedback to the circadian system.

Common zeitgebers include exercise, sleep, and food, but light provides the most potent feedback. The common pathogenesis underlying the extrinsic circadian rhythm disorders is a temporary misalignment between the circadian rhythm and the local time, often exacerbated by inappropriately timed light and activity patterns. The pacemaker activity of the SCN is normally synchronized to the light/dark cycle. The circadian phase can alternatively be ahead of the local light/dark cycle, termed advanced, or behind the local day/night cycle, termed delayed.

Light mediates circadian pacemaker activity by acting on intrinsically photosensitive retinal ganglion cells. Light exposure can appropriately induce phase shifts to adjust the circadian rhythm to local time or new social obligations but can also create disorder in the circadian cycle, with consequent effects on physiology and neurocognitive performance. The population worldwide is aging so it is noteworthy that the ability to tolerate circadian phase misalignment diminishes with increasing age.[2]

The entrained circadian rhythm is vital to physical activity and metabolic, gastrointestinal, and central nervous system homeostasis, with

Disclosure: The authors have no conflicts of interest to report. Funding sources include Roger Williams Medical Center, Boston University, Internal Research Grant unrelated to this article (Dr R.E. Weir) and National Institute of Health, grants unrelated to this article (Dr C.C. Hagen).
[a] Sleep Disorders Program, Portland VA Medical Center, Oregon Health and Science University, CR-139, 3181 Southwest Sam Jackson Road, Portland, OR 97239, USA; [b] Sleep Disorders Program, Oregon Health and Science University, CR-139, 3181 Southwest Sam Jackson Road, Portland, OR 97239, USA
* Corresponding author.
E-mail address: hagench@ohsu.edu

Sleep Med Clin 9 (2014) 561–570
http://dx.doi.org/10.1016/j.jsmc.2014.08.011

abnormalities associated with even short-term circadian malalignment. Examples of the adverse effect of extrinsic circadian alignment on these systems in recent studies include the control of blood sugar, consequent pancreatic insulin production, blood pressure, intimal blood vessel thickness, immune function, and psychological mood and cognitive function.[3,4]

Ambient light levels contribute to the cause of circadian misalignment in shift work and jet lag, and this can also be seen seasonally, in winter months, when lower ambient light exposure is frequently associated with higher population suicide rates and seasonally acquired depression, because a healthy balanced circadian rhythm is essential to normal function on multiple levels ranging from cellular function to gross neurocognitive function.

Poor seasonal or ambient light can prolong the time to adapt to either transmeridian travel or shift work. Symptoms of extrinsic circadian disorders are similar to those of other sleep disorders, namely sleepiness, fatigue, poor or irritable moods, or cognitive inefficiency. Misalignment and the secondary effects are usually temporary and reversed over a period of days to weeks, given sufficient opportunity to recuperate and reentrain. Jet lag and shift work are common acquired circadian rhythm abnormalities resulting from behaving independently from the endogenous circadian rhythm.

JET LAG

In 2013, 29.0 million US travelers visited overseas markets, an increase of 2% from 2012.[5] Most of these trips crossed more than 3 time zones. Many travelers experience the effects of jet lag induced by the mismatch in circadian phase and activity level as they move through time zones at a rate too rapid for normal adaptation to occur. Jet lag arises when the slow innate adaptation present for changes in seasonal ambient light is not immediately able to keep up with rapid circadian phase shifts across different time zones.

The greater the number of time zones crossed, the greater the risk of developing symptoms such as hypersomnia during the period of desired wakefulness or wakefulness and insomnia during the period of desired sleep. Additional fatigue associated with air travel can arise from abrupt change of sleep patterns to reach the airport, change to mealtimes, the stress of travel, and dehydration or low oxygen tension, which can arise during flights. These adverse symptomatic effects are often in addition to baseline sleep deprivation.

In 2010, it was estimated that 30% of the US population had 6 hours sleep or less.[6] Geographic location, distance traveled, duration of time spent in travel, and social obligations at the destination affect the adjustment to local time as ambient light conditions vary. The timing of social obligations at the destination may exacerbate or alleviate the change in time zones. For example, a morning-type retiree traveling 6 hours ahead from Miami, Florida, to Barcelona, Spain, might have little to no change in dinner time and bedtime at the destination relative to the origin. In contrast, traveling just half this distance 3 hours ahead from San Francisco to New York for a 7 AM business meeting could have a large effect on wake time, breakfast time, and morning alertness relative to behavior at origin.

Because most people have an evening tendency, or more easily delayed circadian rhythm, people taking flights in an easterly (earlier) direction are more prone to circadian rhythm symptoms than those traveling in a westerly (later) direction. It has long been recognized that in populations of people this adaptation to jet lag is more rapid when traveling westward, although genetic variability may be a significant factor in interindividual variability, with morning types adapting more readily to eastward travel and evening types adapting more readily to westward travel.[6]

Diagnosis of Jet Lag Disorder

The evaluation for jet lag disorder may be summarized as follows:

1. Diagnosis is made by history.
2. Tests to confirm the diagnosis of jet lag are unnecessary.
3. Tests to identify comorbid sleep disorders may be necessary.
4. Sleep logs or actigraphy can help detect insufficient sleep syndrome.
5. Polysomnography or home apnea testing should be considered if pertinent apnea symptoms are present and sleep complaints persist despite an adequate period within the same time zone.
6. Multiple sleep latency test (MSLT) may be appropriate if hypersomnia and ancillary symptoms of narcolepsy are present, although MSLT should be avoided if there has been recent transmeridian travel because of risk of false-positives from disordered circadian rhythm.

International Classification of Sleep Disorders (ICSD)-3 Diagnostic Criteria for Jet Lag Disorder are shown in **Box 1**.

Box 1
ICSD-3 diagnostic criteria for jet lag disorder

The following 3 criteria must be present:

1. Insomnia or excessive daytime sleepiness and reduced total sleep time associated with crossing 2 or more time zones.
2. Cognitive or somatic symptoms (impaired function, malaise, gastrointestinal complaints) within 2 days of travel.
3. Not better explained by another cause.

From American Academy of Sleep Medicine. International classification of sleep disorders. 3rd edition. Darien (IL): American Academy of Sleep Medicine; 2014; with permission.

Case Example of Jet Lag Without Jet Lag Disorder

A 62-year-old male commercial airline pilot presents with chronic routine transmeridian international and domestic travel resulting in a combination of continuous jet lag and shift work. He reports being naturally resilient throughout his adulthood, recalling rigorous physical and academic military training that was intentionally distributed around the clock amid chronic sleep deprivation in order to identify resilient pilots for the military. He reports a perception of not developing sleepiness, and never having difficulty with insomnia. Average total sleep time per 24-hour period remains within normal limits and all symptoms of sleepiness, impairment, or insomnia were denied. His Epworth score was 2 out of 24, with 2 points because of a moderate chance dozing off if laying down to rest in the afternoon when circumstances permit. Given the risks caused by being a professional pilot, multiple potential sleep disorders that could compromise ability to stay awake and the problem of secondary gain that affect patients' willingness to admit symptoms of sleepiness, a Maintenance of Wakefulness test was completed and confirmed zero epochs of sleep in all naps. Despite severely disturbed sleep/wake pattern, this pilot does not meet ICSD-3 criteria for either shift work or jet lag because he maintains adequate total sleep time per 24-hour period and has no evidence of sleepiness or insomnia. The reason that 60% of shift workers are resilient and do not develop shift work disorder remains unclear. Factors may include variability in neural metabolism, adenosine, cholinergic function, activity in the reticular activating system, or balance of activity within other regions promoting wake and sleep. He has comorbid sleep apnea and uses continuous positive airway pressure (CPAP) for 100% of his sleep. This CPAP permits depiction of his sleep/wake pattern over time (**Fig. 1**). Gray bars indicate time in bed using CPAP. The complete disorganization of his rest/activity cycle results from continuous transmeridian travel and relative shift work.

SHIFT WORK DISORDER

Shift workers play a vital role in a 24-hour society. Night shift workers experience circadian rhythm misalignment when occupational shifts require workers to be awake out of phase with local day/night cycles when local populations tend to sleep. Shift work often results in sleep deprivation in addition to circadian misalignment.

Emerging evidence raises concern about associated health risks of chronic shift work. Epidemiologic studies of shift workers have shown higher rates of cardiovascular disease, obesity, and breast cancer.[7] Newer studies show the induction of pathologic states[8,9] by either the misalignment of circadian cycles or the deprivation of sleep in healthy human research subjects.[4] Sleep deprivation may further exacerbate the increased risk for depression that seems to arise from circadian misalignment.

Diagnosis of Shift Work Disorder

The evaluation for shift work disorder may be summarized as follows:

1. Diagnosed by history combined with sleep log/actigraphy detailing presence/severity of disordered sleep/wake pattern.
2. Tests to identify comorbid sleep disorders that exacerbate shift work disorder symptoms or increase susceptibility to shift work disorder may be necessary.
3. Sleep logs or actigraphy are useful in identifying insufficient sleep syndrome or inadequate sleep hygiene.
4. Consider polysomnography or home apnea testing if pertinent apnea symptoms are present and sleep complaints persist, despite 6 weeks or more of stable sleep/wake pattern.
5. Consider MSLT if hypersomnia and ancillary symptoms of narcolepsy are present, although the test should be avoided in patients with recent shift work history; disordered circadian rhythms cause false-positives.
6. Testing timing of endogenous melatonin secretion could be helpful, but is not commonly available or commonly covered by insurance plans at this time.
7. Maintenance of Wakefulness Test (MWT) may be required if concern for safety in high-risk

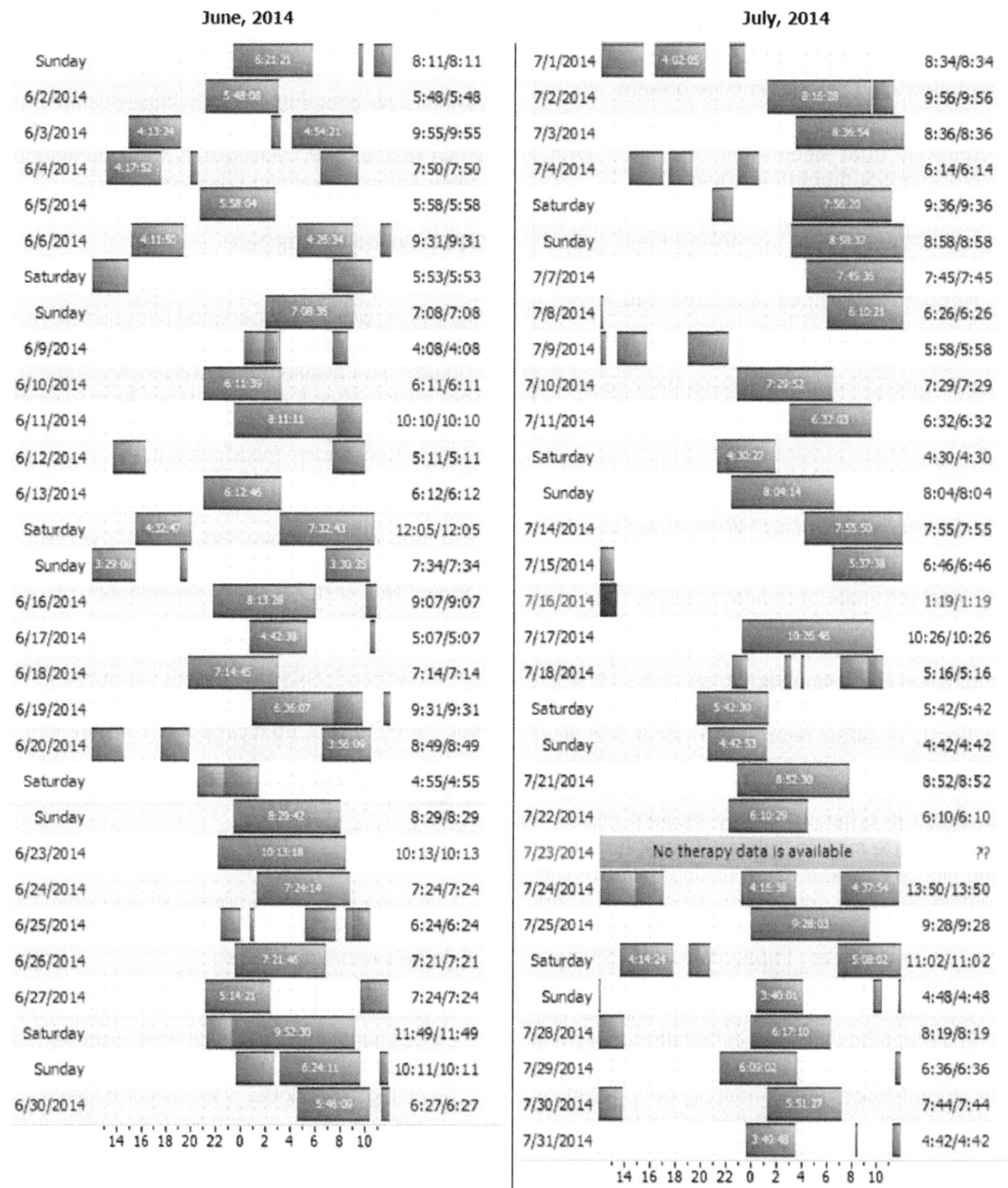

Fig. 1. A 62-year-old pilot with an irregular sleep/wake schedule caused by frequent transmeridian travel and shift work. Nearly perfect CPAP compliance permits identification of sleep/wake cycle, with shaded bars representing time spent sleeping on CPAP.

professions (eg, pilots, ship captains, professional drivers).

ICSD-3 diagnostic criteria for shift work disorder are shown in **Box 2**.

Case Example of Shift Work Disorder

A 60-year-old ship captain developed worsening insomnia and sleepiness after years of prolonged high-frequency shift work of 6 hours on, 6 hours off (**Fig. 2**). His complaints persisted after a prolonged period of time permitted to sleep with a regular sleep/wake schedule. Although originally tolerating this polyphasic sleep schedule of 6 hours working, 6 hours off, alternating for weeks and months at a time, he eventually developed intolerance to this schedule as he aged.

The reason why 40% of shift workers develop shift work disorder remains unclear. The schedule in this case is unusual in that he had a high-

Box 2
ICSD-3 diagnostic criteria for shift work disorder

All 4 of the following criteria must be present:

1. Insomnia or excessive daytime sleepiness and reduced total sleep time associated with a work schedule requiring wake during the usual time for sleep.
2. Symptoms present and associated with shift work schedule for 3 months or more.
3. Sleep log and actigraphy for a continuous period of at least 14 days shows a disordered sleep/wake pattern.
4. Not better explained by other causes.

From American Academy of Sleep Medicine. International classification of sleep disorders. 3rd edition. Darien (IL): American Academy of Sleep Medicine; 2014; with permission.

frequency shift of 6 hours on and 6 hours off, which leads to a polyphasic sleep pattern because all of his needed sleep cannot be contained in any single 6-hour period off work (time is also needed for meals, free time, and so forth). Recent research suggests that a polyphasic sleep pattern or segmented pattern like this in animal models may speed entrainment of the circadian rhythm. In this case, the patient not only had shift work, but had shift work disorder caused by the reduced time for sleep and development of both sleepiness and insomnia at disadvantageous times.

The ideal treatment plan for this case included:

1. Advocacy and letters on the patient's behalf to obtain a healthier and more sustainable work schedule.
2. Continuation of CPAP treatment to make available sleep as efficient as possible.
3. Modafinil as needed, timed during wake intervals.
4. Consideration of a short-acting low-dose hypnotic such as zaleplon 5 mg for intervals with sleep opportunity of 4 to 6 hours. This option increases the risk of impairment or intoxication during wake hours if not tolerated or not cleared rapidly enough and should thus be done cautiously and only continued if clearly improving alertness and function during periods of wake.

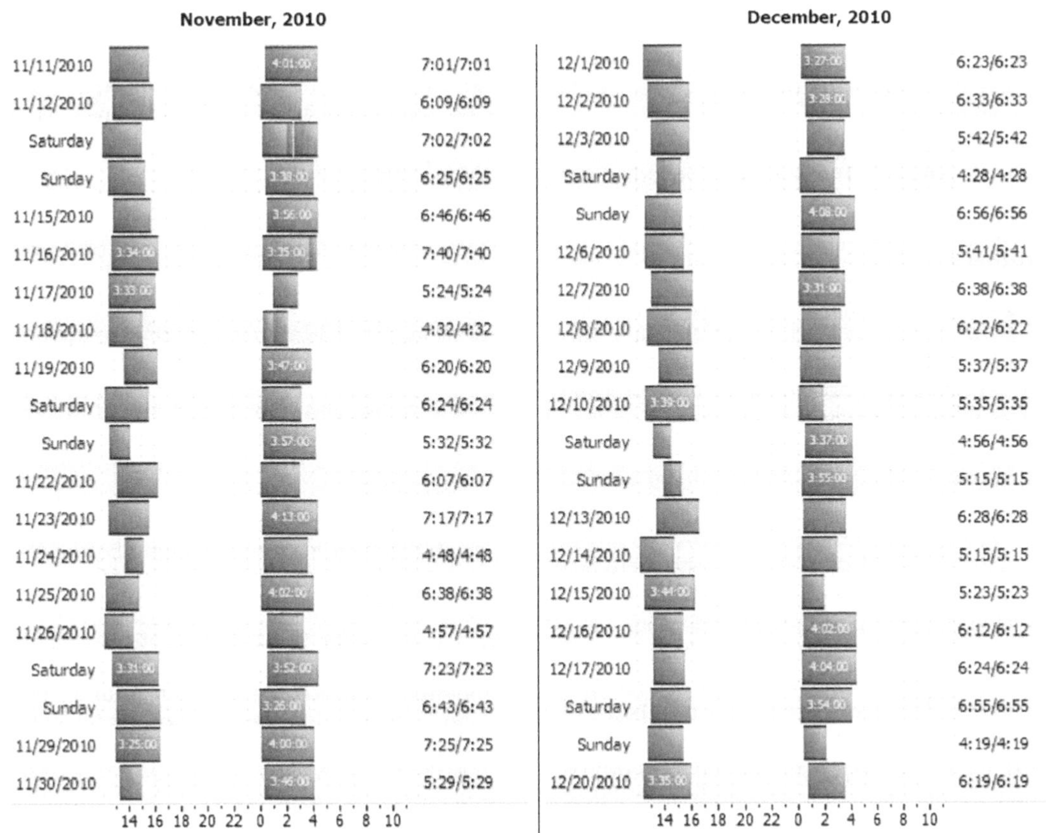

Fig. 2. A 60-year-old ship captain with long-term high-frequency shift work. Perfect CPAP compliance permits identification of sleep/wake cycle, with shaded bars representing time spent sleeping on CPAP.

TREATMENT STRATEGIES FOR JET LAG AND SHIFT WORK DISORDER

The tools used to treat jet lag and shift work disorder are similar and are reviewed together here. The challenge facing physicians is to augment the circadian adaptation and recovery to enable modern patients to optimize their functioning within their new circadian environment, using tolerable techniques that are compatible with lifestyle demands and minimizing the impact of these disorders on health and wellbeing. On a larger scale, population health and function have impacts on occupational safety rates, the efficiency of key services operating outside regular hours, economic productivity, global trade, and international politics, because modern communication and business increasingly extend across traditional geographic boundaries and time zones.

Reentrainment strategies recruit innate, clock-setting mechanisms that fine-tune the circadian system to compensate for the difference between the intrinsic clock (a little more than 24 hours) and the seasonal variances in the solar day (changes in season or latitude). These treatments are in 4 common areas: phototherapy, melatonin supplementation, stimulating medications, or sedating medications. Prevention or attenuation can be attempted by prophylactic circadian phase shifting in advance of travel or modified sleep habits amid shift work.

Key treatment points for jet lag disorder are shown in **Boxes 3–5**. Those for shift work disorder are shown in **Box 6**.

Phototherapy

Jet lag

Timing of phototherapy, whether natural or artificial, is crucial to resetting the circadian clock and is codependent on the number of time zones crossed and the direction of travel to the destination (see **Fig. 1**). Exposure of light in the morning shifts the circadian clock earlier and exposure in the evening shifts the circadian clock later. This timing principle is applied to achieve the intended circadian correction.[10] In the early hours of the morning there is a shift in the timing point when light stimulus is advancing, to a timing point that is delaying.

An aide memoire for morning light exposure after short journeys is "Less for west, and the opposite for east". This rule is reversed once 8 hours of time zones have been crossed, because the timing at dusk local time maybe interpreted as dawn by the new arrival. Thus after 8 hours of time zones have been crossed the general recommendation is to reverse the less-for-west rule when referring to morning light exposure.

Box 3
Jet lag disorder treatment key points

1. Most people tolerate and adapt to westward travel more easily than eastward travel.
2. Greater number of time zones crossed typically results in greater symptom severity and duration.
3. Appropriately timed melatonin can hasten adaptation to jet lag.
4. Appropriately timed bright light can hasten adaptation to jet lag.
5. Conservative measures include maintaining adequate time for sleep before departure and using ear plugs, and eye masks may help avoid unnecessary sleep loss.
6. Hypnotic medications can be used to assist with sleep at destination.
7. Caffeine and short daytime naps improve vigilance at destination.
8. Limit naps to short durations and avoid evening caffeine at destination to promote better sleep at night.

People might also help achieve entrainment by avoiding light exposure or by wearing blue light–blocking sunglasses at the end of the day opposite to that in which light treatment is recommended. Eating should be timed with local meal times because this may also help travelers entrain to the local time zone.[11]

Bright light for jet lag Although durations of published experimental exposures to light vary

Box 4
Eastward travel: light and melatonin treatment key points

1. Bright morning light earlier than habitual wake time for the mornings before departure and on arrival at destination hastens adaptation.
2. Melatonin administered 4 to 6 hours before habitual bedtime for 3 to 5 nights before departure then at bedtime on arrival hastens adaptation to eastward travel.
3. If travel is for few days and social circumstances permit, maintain regular sleep/wake pattern consistent with home routine (ie, go to bed and wake up 3 hours later than usual while traveling from west to east coast in the United States).
4. Greater number of time zones crossed typically results in greater symptom severity and duration.

Box 5
Westward travel: light and melatonin treatment key points

1. Melatonin administered in the early morning hours before departure might have a benefit for westward travel, although further research is needed for confirmation.
2. Late night bright light exposure promotes a delay in circadian rhythm to more westerly time zone.
3. For short duration trips when circumstances permit, maintain a regular sleep/wake pattern consistent with home time zone (ie, go to bed and wake up at a clock time 3 hours earlier than usual while traveling from west to east coast in the United States).
4. Greater number of time zones crossed typically results in greater symptom severity and duration.

widely, one such study was a simulated easterly journey in which sleep schedule was shifted earlier by 1 hour a day for 3 days. Subjects were divided into 3 groups, then on awakening exposed to light of greater than 3000 lux for 3.5 hours continuously, or 30 minutes intermittently (on then off), or to the natural ambient dim light of less than 60 lux. The average dim-light melatonin onset (DLMO) phase advances in the continuous bright light, intermittent bright light, and dim-light groups were 2.1, 1.5, and 0.6 hours, respectively.[12] Other studies have shown beneficial findings after simulated westerly travel correction.[13] It is likely that natural daylight, when present, is the ideal source of light, although artificial light protocols may permit more flexibility to work around social obligations, schedules, and exposure to light when ambient light is inadequate or inaccessible.[14,15]

Use of light for shift work

Bright light exposure during night shifts can improve alertness via its direct alerting effect in addition to the circadian phase shifting effects of light.[16]

Short naps may also be useful for reducing the decrements in night shift alertness.[17]

These interventions do not overcome reductions in alertness occurring in the early hours of the morning.

Box 6
Shift work disorder treatment key points

Lifestyle changes

- Adjust timing of exposure to daylight
- Maximizing overlap of sleep period for nights on versus nights off may improve quality of sleep
- Advocate for healthier and more stable shifts

Sleep hygiene

- Help patients identify their chronotypes and encourage work shifts that fit this natural preference
- Evaluate for and treat any insufficient sleep syndrome
- Change timing of daily routines to permit a regular sleep/wake schedule 7 nights per week
- Strategically scheduling naps may help in addition to consistency of sleep timing **(Fig. 3)**

Light

- Synchronize body clock by exposing safe levels of intense, bright light for brief durations at strategic times of day as appropriate to patients' shifts
- Patients should use blue light–blocking glasses during drive home after night shifts

Medications

- Taking melatonin at precise times may help stabilize the circadian phase in accordance with desired shift work schedules
- Hypnotics may improve the ability to sleep out of phase with the circadian phase
- Modafinil is approved by the US Food and Drug Administration for treatment of shift work disorder
- Patients should avoid self-medication with drugs or alcohol
- Counsel patients to prevent risks of impaired decision making, and avoid operation of machinery or vehicles while drowsy

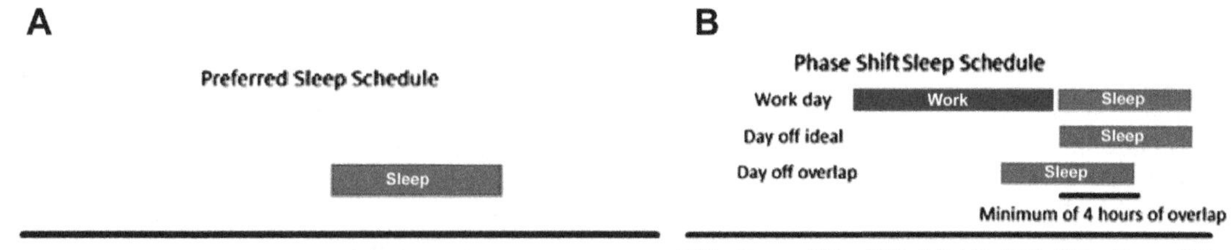

Fig. 3. Maximizing the consistency of sleep despite shift work. (*A*) A common evening preferred sleep schedule. (*B*) Sleep schedules for nonwork days. The top and center schedules are ideal sleep schedules at the same time for both days on and days off, 7 days per week despite shift work. The bottom schedule shows a compromised 4-hour overlap schedule that permits at least 4 hours of consistently timed sleep every night of the week with an additional 4 hours earlier on days off and 4 hours later on work days.

Circadian rhythm can be advanced by exposing people to bright light in the morning, and can be delayed by bright light exposure in the late afternoon/evening. By varying the timing of light exposure, natural or otherwise, circadian rhythm can be adjusted to optimize shift work.

Blue light–blocking glasses or strict avoidance of light during the hours leading up to sleep or intended for sleep can improve entrainment of the circadian rhythm to the desired phase.

Melatonin Supplements

Melatonin is usually secreted by the pineal gland for 10 to 12 hours every night and levels in the saliva are one method used to determine degree of circadian entrainment, another being minimal body temperature. Melatonin secretion is also controlled by the circadian system, and coincides with the darkness section of the cycle. Although melatonin is not approved by the US Food and Drug Administration (FDA), when it is supplemented in the evening before endogenous secretion it has the effect of resetting the body clock to an earlier time. This feedback loop is thought to be mediated by melatonin receptors found on the suprachiasmatic nuclei.[18]

Of secondary importance is a hypnotic effect occurring with higher doses, typically administered at a time closer to the desired onset of sleep.

The use of melatonin was reviewed in a 2002 Cochrane Review[19] on subjective ratings of well-being, daytime tiredness, sleep onset, sleep quality, psychological functioning, duration of return to normal, and indicators of circadian rhythms measured. Nine of the 10 randomized trials of airline passengers, airline staff, or military personnel given oral melatonin decreased jet lag from flights when crossing 5 or more time zones, compared with placebo or other medication, when taken close to the target destination (10 PM to midnight). Again, reentrainment to advance sleep (and wake time) was intrinsically more difficult than that of delaying sleep onset and wake time.

Melatonin use is particularly recommended in adults crossing more than 5 time zones, especially those traveling in an easterly destination. Travelers crossing only 2 to 4 time zones may still benefit from taking melatonin if needed based on patient history or reaction to travel because jet lag symptoms are more likely in patients with a previous history of difficulty tolerating jet lag.

Doses of 0.5 mg to 5 mg were similarly effective; however, a 2-mg slow-release dose was less effective, suggesting either that the surge in melatonin concentration might be important or that spillover onto the delay zone of the phase response curve to melatonin may need to be avoided. In 2 studies the number needed to treat was 2. Attempts to shift the circadian phase in the direction of the destination pattern for 3 to 5 days before traveling may hasten adaptation and lessen the severity of jet lag.

Melatonin metabolism is via liver P450 2C9 (cytochrome P2C9 [CYP2C9]), which shows polymorphism and mutations, and is subject to induction by rifampin, phenobarbital, and dexamethasone. P450 2C9 (CYP2C9) also metabolizes S-warfarin, and melatonin therefore has the potential to interfere with warfarin metabolism.[20] Current evidence concerning the effect on epilepsy is conflicting, and there is no clear contraindication to melatonin use in patients with epilepsy.[21] Routine melatonin pharmacology and toxicology requires further study, and improved quality control would be beneficial for the manufacture of this supplement, which is not regulated by the FDA.

Melatonin for shift work

Three milligrams have been shown to advance circadian rhythm by significantly larger amounts than placebo controls; however, in the hours between melatonin ingestion and bed, melatonin caused sleepiness and performance decrements, prompting investigators to suggest lower treatment doses.[22]

Typical current doses of 0.5 mg are administered a few hours before desired sleep onset;

furthermore, the Cochrane Review did not detect significant differences in the level of effect observed with different doses, suggesting that lower doses are probably adequate without unnecessary side effects, although some debate remains about the optimum phase-shifting dose of melatonin for shift work and jet lag.

Overlap Schedule Versus Full Entrainment for Shift Work

Although full entrainment provides optimal performance, it has the disadvantage of limiting activities during periods of days off.

Different degrees of circadian rhythm entrainment have been studied in simulated night workers and the performance at different levels of circadian entrainment measured. A compromise between full adaptation is shown to produce good performance measures by delaying the sleepiest circadian time out of the night work period. This time is defined to occur approximately 7 hours after DLMO, and can be assessed by measuring melatonin in the saliva. DLMO occurring in the partially adapted night shift group occurs between 0130 and 0500 hours. On days off this occurs toward the end of the sleep cycle for partially entrained workers. This overlap schedule balances enhanced social function on days off with improved sleep quality and performance across the week. It does so by increasing time awake during the day on days off while restricting the change in sleep period from night to night relative to workers that alternate sleeping during the day and sleeping at night.

Such partially entrained adjustment periods produced favorable performance compared with non–circadian-entrained groups and similar to fully entrained circadian patterns. Individual optimal patterns may vary but this compromise may be useful when advising patients undertaking night shift work.[23]

Pharmacologic Approaches to Sleepiness

Sleep deprivation increases low-frequency electroencephalogram (EEG) activity in wakefulness, non-rapid eye movement (NREM) sleep, and rapid eye movement (REM) sleep.[24,25] High EEG slow wave activity or delta activity (spectral power within ~ 0.5–4.5 Hz) is characteristic of deep NREM sleep and an established marker of sleep homeostasis.[26] This activity increases after sleep deprivation.

Caffeine is a competitive adenosine A1 and A2A receptor antagonist and, on EEG studies, caffeine reduces theta activity (5–8 Hz) in waking and slow wave activity in NREM and REM sleep, and enhances spindle frequency activity (~11–15 Hz) and beta oscillations (>16 Hz) in NREM recovery sleep. These findings suggest that caffeine attenuates the prolonged wake-induced buildup of sleep need.[27]

Caffeine can improve function and lessen severity of symptoms and should be timed appropriately to permit strategic naps with durations of 30 minutes to 1 hour. Longer naps may delay reentrainment but may be more appropriate according to individual timetable demands for work or jet lag.

Ker and colleagues[28] conducted a Cochrane Review of 13 trials from 2008 to 2010. Two trials measured errors made and cognitive performance using neuropsychological testing methods. The review concluded that caffeine might, within normal levels, be an effective intervention for improving performance in shift workers. There were significantly reduced numbers of errors compared with placebo, with improved concept formation, reasoning, memory, orientation, attention, and perception. Although one trial comparing caffeine with napping found significantly fewer errors in the caffeine group compared with the nap group, overall there was no difference between caffeine and nap, bright light, or modafinil interventions.

Modafinil

In contrast with the adenosine receptor antagonist caffeine, modafinil induced no changes in slow wave sleep and EEG slow wave activity in NREM sleep after sleep deprivation. This finding suggests that modafinil leaves NREM sleep rebound unaffected after prolonged wakefulness. Modafinil is approved by the FDA for shift work sleep disorder and persistent hypersomnia despite obstructive sleep apnea-hypopnea syndrome.[29] Caffeine and amphetamine were shown to be more wakefulness promoting on the Stanford Sleepiness Test Score than modafinil. EEG studies indicate caffeine, amphetamine, and modafinil to all be theta wave reducing but only modafinil to be alpha wave promoting during wakefulness as well as theta wave increasing during sleep.[30]

The usual prescribed dosage for shift work disorder is 200 mg once during required wakefulness, although doses up to 400 mg per 24-hour period may be used in other conditions such as sleep apnea or narcolepsy. Modafinil is not approved for the treatment of children because of the occurrence of severe allergic reactions, including Stephens-Johnson. Armodafinil has a similar half-life to modafinil but seems to have a longer duration of higher concentrations caused by a steady decline in concentration as opposed to a bimodal reduction of modafinil, which may be caused by modafinil's inclusion of 2 enantiomers. Armodafinil at a dose of 150 mg per day increased wakefulness after simulated eastbound travel through 6 time zones in 143 participants, compared with 142 controls, and was generally well tolerated.[31]

REFERENCES

1. Solt LA, Wang Y, Banerjee S, et al. Regulation of circadian behaviour and metabolism by synthetic REV-ERB agonists. Nature 2012;485(7396):62–8.
2. Sack RL. Clinical practice. Jet lag. N Engl J Med 2010;362(5):440–7.
3. Shea SA. Obesity and pharmacologic control of the body clock. N Engl J Med 2012;367(2):175–8.
4. Scheer FA, Hilton MF, Mantzoros CS, et al. Adverse metabolic and cardiovascular consequences of circadian misalignment. Proc Natl Acad Sci U S A 2009;106(11):4453–8.
5. Available at: http://travel.trade.gov/outreachpages/download_data_table/2013_Outbound_Analysis.pdf. Accessed July 27, 2014.
6. Aschoff J, Hoffmann K, Pohl H, et al. Re-entrainment of circadian rhythms after phase-shifts of the Zeitgeber. Chronobiologia 1975;2(1):23–78.
7. Stevens RG, Brainard GC, Blask DE, et al. Breast cancer and circadian disruption from electric lighting in the modern world. CA Cancer J Clin 2014; 64(3):207–18.
8. Buxton OM, Cain SW, O'Connor SP, et al. Adverse metabolic consequences in humans of prolonged sleep restriction combined with circadian disruption. Sci Transl Med 2012;4(129):129ra43.
9. Monteggia LM, Kavalali ET. Circadian rhythms: depression brought to light. Nature 2012;491(7425): 537–8.
10. Khalsa SB, Jewett ME, Cajochen C, et al. A phase response curve to single bright light pulses in human subjects. J Physiol 2003;549(Pt 3):945–52.
11. Herxheimer A, Waterhouse J. The prevention and treatment of jet lag. BMJ 2003;326(7384):296–7.
12. Burgess HJ, Crowley SJ, Gazda CJ, et al. Preflight adjustment to eastward travel: 3 days of advancing sleep with and without morning bright light. J Biol Rhythms 2003;18(4):318–28.
13. Boulos Z, Macchi MM, Sturchler MP, et al. Light visor treatment for jet lag after westward travel across six time zones. Aviat Space Environ Med 2002;73(10): 953–63.
14. Morrissette DA. Twisting the night away: a review of the neurobiology, genetics, diagnosis, and treatment of shift work disorder. CNS Spectr 2013; 18(Suppl 1):45–53 [quiz: 54].
15. Sack RL, Auckley D, Auger RR, et al. Circadian rhythm sleep disorders: part I, basic principles, shift work and jet lag disorders. An American Academy of Sleep Medicine review. Sleep 2007;30(11):1460–83.
16. Campbell SS, Terman M, Lewy AJ, et al. Light treatment for sleep disorders: consensus report. V. Age-related disturbances. J Biol Rhythms 1995;10(2): 151–4.
17. Schweitzer PK, Randazzo AC, Stone K, et al. Laboratory and field studies of naps and caffeine as practical countermeasures for sleep-wake problems associated with night work. Sleep 2006;29(1):39–50.
18. Dubocovich M, Benloucif S, Masana MI. Melatonin receptors in the mammalian suprachiasmatic nucleus. Behav Brain Res 1996;73(1–2):141–7.
19. Herxheimer A, Petrie Keith J. Melatonin for the prevention and treatment of jet lag. Cochrane Database Syst Rev 2002;(2):CD001520.
20. Zhou SF, Zhou ZW, Yang LP, et al. Substrates, inducers, inhibitors and structure-activity relationships of human cytochrome P450 2C9 and implications in drug development. Curr Med Chem 2009;16(27): 3480–675.
21. Jain S, Besag FM. Does melatonin affect epileptic seizures? Drug Saf 2013;36(4):207–15.
22. Crowley SJ, Eastman CI. Melatonin in the afternoons of a gradually advancing sleep schedule enhances the circadian rhythm phase advance. Psychopharmacology (Berl) 2013;225(4):825–37.
23. Smith MR, Fogg LF, Eastman CI. A compromise circadian phase position for permanent night work improves mood, fatigue, and performance. Sleep 2009;32(11):1481–9.
24. Lim J, Dinges DF. Sleep deprivation and vigilant attention. Ann N Y Acad Sci 2008;1129:305–22.
25. Goel N, Rao H, Durmer JS, et al. Neurocognitive consequences of sleep deprivation. Semin Neurol 2009;29(4):320–39.
26. Borbely AA, Baumann F, Brandeis D, et al. Sleep deprivation: effect on sleep stages and EEG power density in man. Electroencephalogr Clin Neurophysiol 1981;51(5):483–95.
27. Bodenmann S, Landolt HP. Effects of modafinil on the sleep EEG depend on Val158Met genotype of COMT. Sleep 2010;33(8):1027–35.
28. Ker K, Edwards PJ, Felix LM, et al. Caffeine for the prevention of injuries and errors in shift workers. Cochrane Database Syst Rev 2010;(5):CD008508.
29. Kesselheim AS, Myers JA, Solomon DH, et al. The prevalence and cost of unapproved uses of top-selling orphan drugs. PLoS One 2012;7(2):e31894.
30. Schmidt C, Collette F, Leclercq Y, et al. Homeostatic sleep pressure and responses to sustained attention in the suprachiasmatic area. Science 2009;324(5926): 516–9.
31. Rosenberg RP, Bogan RK, Tiller JM, et al. A phase 3, double-blind, randomized, placebo-controlled study of armodafinil for excessive sleepiness associated with jet lag disorder. Mayo Clin Proc 2010;85(7): 630–8.

Poor Sleep with Age

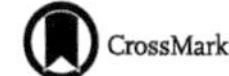

Vikas Jain, MD, FAASM, CCSH

KEYWORDS

• Sleep evaluation • Children • Adolescence • Adults • Elderly

KEY POINTS

- Understanding normal changes that occur with respect to sleep during the aging process, including changes to sleep architecture as well as napping patterns, is important when evaluating sleep complaints.
- A multidisciplinary approach to the clinical evaluation of sleep complaints, including diagnostic questions, pertinent systems during examination, and various studies, is recommended.
- Understanding the diagnosis and management of common sleep disorders that are prevalent in different stages of life can help with narrowing the possible differential diagnoses.

INTRODUCTION

Sleep is an essential biological function and is dynamic process that has psychological and physiologic effects throughout the lifespan. The symptoms that are frequently present as well as the sleep disorders that often manifest vary as an individual ages. During childhood, behavioral sleep issues often contribute to poor sleep. As an individual moves into adolescence and there is a physiologic phase delay in sleep timing, circadian rhythm disorders are more likely. During adulthood, there is a predominance of insomnia complaints as well as a higher prevalence of breathing and movement disorders. In the elderly, a large contributing factor to poor sleep is commonly polypharmacy as well as the high prevalence of medical and psychiatric comorbidities. Sleep complaints, when persistent, can result in daytime sleepiness, which can lead to morbidity in elderly patients, such as impaired cognition, delirium, disorientation, dementia, as well as increase the risk of falls. Another concern is the bidirectional relationships between sleep disorders and many medical disorders. Patients with sleep disorders are often more likely to develop cardiovascular and cerebrovascular disorders, and individuals with a history of these disorders are often at a higher risk of developing sleep disorders. During this review, the evaluation of sleep complaints is discussed along with presentation and management options of common sleep disorders encountered in the 4 major stages of life mentioned earlier.

SLEEP CHANGES WITH AGING

Sleep Architecture

When evaluating sleep complaints, it is first important to understand normal age-related changes that can occur in sleep parameters. Ohayon and colleagues[1] conducted a meta-analysis based on data from 3577 subjects aged 5 years to 102 years and demonstrated that several changes occur in both sleep architecture as well as sleep parameters throughout the lifespan.[1] These changes include a reduction in total sleep time, sleep efficiency, and slow-wave sleep as well as an increase in wake after sleep onset as an individual ages (**Table 1**). There is also a reduction in REM sleep percentages, whereas the percentage of stage N1 and stage N2 sleep increases. Given that the electrical resistance of the skull increases with age, it is important to note that the reduction in slow-wave sleep may result from a reduction in the electroencephalogram amplitude rather than a true reduction in slow-wave frequency. When only older adults (aged >60 years) were evaluated, only sleep efficiency was found to decline, whereas the

The author has nothing to disclose.

Sleep Medicine, 3555 Northwest 58th Street, Suite 310W, Oklahoma City, OK 73112, USA
E-mail address: vikasjainmd@gmail.com

Sleep Med Clin 9 (2014) 571–583
http://dx.doi.org/10.1016/j.jsmc.2014.08.008
1556-407X/14/$ – see front matter

Table 1
Summary of significant sleep changes during the lifespan

	Child to Adolescent	Young Adult to Old Adult	Old Adult to Elderly
Sleep latency	←→	←→	←→
Sleep efficiency	←→	↓	↓
Stage 1 sleep	←→	↑	↑
Stage 2 sleep	↑	↑	↑
Slow-wave sleep	↓	↓	↓
REM sleep	↑	↓	↓
Wake after sleep onset	↓	↑	↑

Child, 5–12 years; adolescent, 13–18 years; young adult, 18–40 years; old adult, 40–60 years; elderly, greater than 60 years. ↓, decrease; ↑, increase; ←→, no change.

Data from Ohayon MM, Carskadon M, Guilleminault C, et al. Meta-analysis of quantitative sleep parameters from childhood to old age in healthy individuals: developing normative sleep values across the human lifespan. Sleep 2004;27:1255–73.

other sleep measures did not reveal any age-related changes. Therefore, it seems that most of the age-related changes in sleep occurs during 19 to 60 years of age. This consideration may be important when determining whether a patient's complaint may be caused by normal aging or is a symptom of an underlying disorder.

Napping

In the newborn, sleep is primarily distributed equally across the day and night. By 6 months of age, an infant has typically developed the ability to sleep through the night. Napping during the day is common in infants and may often last until 3 to 5 years of age. A common misconception regarding sleep in elderly patients is that there is a reduction in the total sleep requirement. Although the duration of sleep during the nocturnal period is reduced, this seems to be offset by an increase in daytime napping. The overall prevalence of daytime napping has been reported to range between 22% and 61%.[2–4] Buysse and coworkers[2] evaluated napping patterns between older (mean age = 78 years) and younger (mean age = 30 years) adults and found that older adults reported taking more naps than their younger counterparts (3.4 naps vs 1.1, respectively). The National Sleep Foundation's 2003 Sleep in America poll on sleep and aging found that 10% of individuals aged between 55 and 64 years reported taking 4 to 7 naps a week, whereas 24% of individuals aged 75 to 84 years reported napping the same frequency.[3] These studies suggest that the prevalence of napping increases with age. When documenting daytime napping, it is important to pay close attention to whether the naps are intentional or unintentional. Napping that is unintentional is more likely to be related to an underlying sleep disorder than planned napping.

Clinical Evaluation of Sleep Complaints

The clinical evaluation of sleep complaints should begin with a comprehensive history and physical examination. The evaluation should include a detailed history and examination, the use of sleep surveys, and objective testing.

Sleep History

When considering sleep complaints in patients, the clinician should gather a comprehensive sleep history (**Box 1**). If need be, it may be important to also obtain history from the patients' spouse, children, parents, bed partner, or caregiver to help to corroborate the patients' sleep complaints. These individuals may also provide useful information regarding sleep complaints that patients may be unaware of, such as snoring or periodic limb movements. The evaluation often begins with the patients' chief complaint. This also often serves to help in the formulation of a differential diagnosis of possible causes for the complaint (**Box 2**).

A detailed account of the patients' sleep schedule should be obtained with information regarding sleep and wake time during the week and on weekends. It is also important to pay attention to the patients' sleep schedule during school versus a holiday in school-aged children and to ask about varying work and sleep schedules in a shift worker. Information about the patients' typical latency to sleep as well as the number and length of awakenings during the night can help to establish baseline sleep efficiency.

If patients have prolonged sleep latency, the clinician should ask how the patients spend this

Box 1
Sleep history

At what time do you go to sleep at night?

At what time do you wake up in the morning?

Do these hours differ on the weekends/days off?

How long does it take you to fall asleep?

Does anyone share the same sleeping space as you (bed partner, children, pets)?

Do you or have you taken any medications to help you fall or stay asleep (prescription vs over the counter)?

Do you wake up in the middle of night? If so, how many times? How long does it take you to fall back asleep?

How many hours do you feel you sleep a night?

Do you feel refreshed when you awaken in the morning?

Do you feel excessively sleepy during the daytime? Do you feel drowsy when you drive? Are there any daytime activities that you are unable to perform because of your sleepiness?

Do you have any difficulty with concentration or memory?

Do you take any naps during the day? If so, how many? For how long do you nap? Do you find your naps to be refreshing?

Questions related to sleep apnea, nocturnal movements, narcolepsy (snoring, witnessed apneas, gasping/choking spells, uncomfortable sensation in legs in the evening with powerful urge to move, bed partner reporting frequent leg kicks or jerking, sleep violence, sleep walking, cataplexy, sleep paralysis, hypnopompic or hypnogogic hallucinations).

Questions related to parasomnias (seizurelike activity, sleep walking, sleep talking, sleep violence, nightmares, night terrors, sleep eating, sleep groaning, head banging).

time, as it may give rise to information regarding the patients' sleep hygiene (watching television, prolonged time in bed, and so forth). If patients have trouble falling asleep, symptoms such as racing thoughts may suggest underlying insomnia or an urge to move the legs may point toward restless legs syndrome (RLS). If patients complain of trouble staying asleep, symptoms such as snoring, gasping, choking, witnessed apneas, morning headaches, nasal congestion, and dry mouth may support a diagnosis of obstructive sleep apnea (OSA). When considering excessive sleepiness during the daytime, special attention should be paid to asking about cataplexy as well as the

Box 2
Chief complaint and possible causes

I cannot fall or stay asleep during the night

Sleep hygiene

Insomnia

Sleep apnea

Restless legs

Medications

Circadian rhythm disorder

I cannot stay awake during the day

Sleep hygiene

Insufficient sleep syndrome

Narcolepsy/idiopathic hypersomnia

Obstructive sleep apnea

Circadian rhythm disorder

Sleep disruption caused by medical disorder

Medications

Strange things occur during my sleep

Seizure disorder

NREM parasomnias

REM parasomnias

Rhythmic movement disorders

Abbreviations: NREM, non-REM; REM, rapid eye movement.

length and restorative nature of daytime naps, as this may support a diagnosis of narcolepsy. Finally, when evaluating unusual behaviors at night, the clinician may consider inquiring about the timing of the events at night. This information may help in differentiating between rapid-eye-movement (REM) and non-REM (NREM) parasomnias. The presence of stereotypical behavior at night may warrant further evaluation for epilepsy.

In the pediatric patient population, it is important to pay close attention to the patients' total sleep duration, as sleep requirements are often beyond the typical 7 to 9 hours seen in adults.[5] Pediatric patients may also often describe atypical symptoms in regard to OSA, as they may often present with hyperactivity and inattention rather than daytime fatigue. In elderly patients, it is also important to pay close attention to the medication history, as polypharmacy is common among this patient population. Many commonly prescribed medications in the elderly can disrupt sleep, including over-the-counter decongestants, corticosteroids, and antidepressants.

Physical Examination

The physical examination of patients can also help to further identify the cause of the patients' complaints. A comprehensive physical examination should be performed, as various findings can help to support the patients' diagnosis (**Table 2**). The examination should include assessment for craniofacial anomalies. In children, there should also be documentation of growth parameters and developmental milestones. Examination of the upper airway may reveal evidence of a narrow upper airway that could contribute to sleep-disordered breathing. Examination of other body systems, such as the cardiovascular, respiratory, or gastrointestinal systems, may reveal evidence of other medical disorders that may contribute to the patients' sleep complaints.

Table 2
Physical examination pearls

Finding	Possible Cause
General	
• Obesity	OSA
Head, Eyes, Ear, Nose, Throat	
• Nose	OSA
○ Nasal valve collapse	
○ Septal deviation	
○ Turbinate hypertrophy	
• Oral	
○ Narrow hard palate	
○ Elongated soft palate/ uvula	
○ Mallampati score	
○ Tonsillar hypertrophy	
• Craniofacial	
○ Maxillary deficiency	
○ Retrognathia	
○ Micrognathia	
• Redundant soft tissue of the palate	
• Retrognathia	
• Mandibular hypoplasia	
Respiratory	
• Expiratory wheezing	Nocturnal asthma
• Kyphoscoliosis	Hypoventilation syndromes
Cardiovascular	
• Fourth heart sound	OSA or central sleep apnea
• Pedal edema	
Abdominal	
• Hepatomegaly	Sleep disruption caused by alcohol abuse
Extremities	
• Joint swelling/ deformity	Sleep disruption caused by arthritis
• Unexplained bruises	Parasomnias
Psychiatric	
• Blunted affect	Depression
• Poor hygiene	

Questionnaires and Diagnostic Testing

During the evaluation of sleep complaints, subjective and objective measurements may also be considered.

A commonly used questionnaire to assess daytime sleepiness is the Epworth Sleepiness Scale, which assesses an individual's likelihood to fall asleep in 8 different scenarios. Patients are asked to rate their probability of dozing as none (0), slight (1), moderate (2), and high (3). These scores are assigned to 8 different scenarios: (1) sitting and reading, (2) watching television, (3) sitting inactive in a public place, (4) riding as a passenger in a car for an hour without a break, (5) lying down to rest in the afternoon when circumstances permit, (6) sitting and talking quietly with someone, (7) sitting quietly after lunch without alcohol, and (8) in a car while stopped in traffic for a few minutes. A total score of 10 or more is typically considered representative of excessive sleepiness.[5] The Pittsburgh Sleep Quality Index (PSQI) is another widely used questionnaire that serves to provide a measure of sleep quality. The PSQI is composed of 19 self-rated questions that are grouped into 7 component scores, each weighted with a score of 0 to 3. These scores are summed to yield a global PSQI score, with higher scores indicating poorer sleep quality.[6] In children, several sleep screening questionnaires, such as the BEARS (Bedtime, Excessive Daytime Sleepiness, Awakening during the Night, Regularity and Duration of Sleep, Snoring) and Children's Sleep Habits Questionnaire, can also assist in the evaluation of sleep complaints.[7,8]

Sleep diaries can also be a useful adjunct to sleep evaluation. Patients should be asked to keep a 2-week log in which they notate their bedtime, sleep latency, frequency and duration of nocturnal awakenings, final awakening, and nap times during the day. An advantage of the sleep diary is that it is not only useful when considering circadian rhythm abnormalities or insomnia but also serves to provide patients with the opportunity to monitor and reflect on their own sleep habits. Wrist-actigraphy is a noninvasive method of monitoring sleep patterns that has been validated and is often performed when considering circadian rhythm disorders.[9]

Polysomnography is an objective tool that can be used to provide confirmatory data during the evaluation of sleep apnea, narcolepsy, periodic limb movement disorder, seizures, and parasomnias. Although polysomnography has been traditionally performed attended in a sleep laboratory, more recently, ambulatory monitoring has been found to be a technically acceptable alternative in both adults and children. The Multiple Sleep Latency Test is a laboratory study designed to measure an individual's tendency to fall asleep. It consists of five 20-minute naps separated by 2-hour intervals during which an individual is instructed to go to sleep and their onset to sleep is documented. A limitation of this testing is that there has been a wide standard deviation in normal controls undergoing testing and that the test has not been validated in both children younger than 8 years and elderly populations.[10] Nonetheless, it is an important tool when considering daytime during the sleep evaluation.

SLEEP DISORDERS ACROSS THE LIFESPAN

Children (0–12 Years of Age)

Prevalence and characteristics of sleep disorders

Studies have reported a prevalence of sleep problems in children ranging from 25% to 50% in preschool-aged children and 20% to 43% in school-aged children.[11–13] In a study by Owens and colleagues,[14] sleep questionnaires were administered to a group of 494 school-aged children in grades kindergarten through fourth as well as their teachers and parents. The most commonly reported parent-defined sleep problems were bedtime resistance and parasomnias with a prevalence of 15.1% and 12.6%, respectively.[14]

Behavioral insomnia of childhood (BIC) is the most common sleep disorder seen in toddlers and preschoolers. The essential diagnostic feature is the report of difficulty falling sleep, staying asleep, or both (**Box 3**). As discussed earlier, as newborns typically have polyphasic sleep, the diagnosis of BIC is not considered until after 6 months of age. BIC generally results from negative sleep associations that can then contribute to either prolonged sleep latency or frequent awakenings at night.[15] In young children with the sleep-onset-association type, behaviors such as rocking or nursing to help the child fall asleep can become learned and, thus, can prevent the child from returning to sleep without the associated stimulus for sleep present during awakenings. Children with the limit-setting type will often use a variety of strategies (asking for a drink, another story, use restroom) to prolong and delay bedtime. These behaviors can result in insufficient sleep duration that can manifest as behavioral symptoms during the day of increased irritability and hyperactivity.

Box 3
Diagnostic criteria of behavioral insomnia of childhood

1. A child's symptoms meet the criteria for insomnia based on parental report or that of other caregivers.
2. The child shows a pattern consistent with either sleep-onset-association type or limit-setting type of insomnia described below:
   a. Sleep-onset-association type includes each of the following:
      i. Falling asleep is an extended process that requires special conditions.
      ii. Sleep-onset associations are highly problematic or demanding.
      iii. In the absence of the associated conditions, sleep onset is significantly delayed or sleep is otherwise disrupted.
      iv. Nighttime awakenings require caregiver intervention for the child to return to sleep.
   b. Limit-setting type includes each of the following:
      i. The individual has difficulty initiating or maintaining sleep.
      ii. The individual stalls or refuses to go to bed at an appropriate time or refuses to return to bed following a nighttime awakening.
      iii. The caregiver demonstrates insufficient or inappropriate limit setting to establish appropriate sleeping behavior in the child.
3. The sleep disturbance is not better explained by another sleep disorder, medical or neurologic disorder, mental disorder, or medication use.

From American Academy of Sleep Medicine. International classification of sleep disorders. In: Sateia M, editor. Diagnostic and coding manual. 3rd edition. Darien (IL): American Academy of Sleep Medicine; 2014. p. 23; with permission.

Parasomnias are undesirable events that occur either during the onset of sleep, during sleep, or during arousals from sleep. Parasomnias are generally seen in either REM or NREM sleep, with NREM parasomnias being more common in children. NREM parasomnias are generally classified into 3 categories: confusional arousals, sleepwalking, and sleep terrors. Clinical features of these 3 categories are summarized in **Table 3**.

Table 3
Clinical features of NREM parasomnias

Clinical Feature	Confusional Arousal	Sleep Terror	Sleep Walking
Age of onset (y)	2–10	2–10	5–10
Frequency	3–4/wk to 1–2/mo	3–4/wk to 1–2/mo	3–4/wk to 1–2/mo
Peak time of occurrence	First third of night sleep	First third of night sleep	First third of night sleep
Ictal behavior	Whimpering, some articulation, sitting up in bed, inconsolable	Screaming, agitation, flushed face, sweating, inconsolable	Walking about the room or house, may be quiet or agitated; unresponsive to verbal commands
Ictal polysomnogram	Slow-wave sleep with rhythmic theta or delta activity	Slow-wave sleep with rhythmic theta or delta activity	Slow-wave sleep with rhythmic theta or delta activity
Duration (min)	10–30	10–20	10–20

Adapted from Kotagal S. Parasomnias of childhood. Curr Opin Pediatr 2008;20:659–65.

A common diagnostic element is that the NREM parasomnias typically occur within the first third of the night, the period of sleep during which there is a higher prevalence of slow-wave sleep activity. Confusional arousals often involve the child whimpering or crying during the episode; however, there is no sweating, flushing, or agitation that is often seen with night terrors. Sleepwalking typically involves ambulation, which can vary from simple events, such as sitting up in bed, to more complex movements, such as walking or running.

Management

BIC and parasomnias in children often can be managed with behavioral interventions. Caregivers should be instructed about creating an appropriate sleep environment and to implement a consistent bedtime routing and sleep schedule. It is important to understand the typical sleep duration requirements in children as mentioned earlier to ensure that an adequate opportunity for sleep is provided.

In BIC, studies have found that behavioral techniques can be used to help resolve the negative association that has been learned.[16] Unmodified extinction involves placing the child in bed at a designated time and then ignoring the child until the next morning. As many parents find it difficult to ignore their child for long periods at a time, graduated extinction is another approach that can be used. This approach involves placing the child in bed at a designated time and then parents are instructed to check on the child at either a fixed or progressively increasing interval until the child falls asleep. If the child continues to have prolonged sleep latency, fading the child's bedtime can help to improve sleep initiation; once the behavior is established, the bedtime can then be advanced by 15 to 30 minutes until the original bedtime goal is reached.

Management of parasomnias should focus on attempting to eliminate the occurrence of events as well as to mitigate the adverse effects of a potential episode. Underlying disorders that may be contributing to the emergence of the parasomnia should be treated. Patients should also be given counseling regarding safety precautions within the home. Emphasis should also be placed on adequate sleep duration, as sleep deprivation can increase parasomnia episodes. If the parasomnia remains problematic, pharmacologic agents, such as benzodiazepines, tricyclic antidepressants and selective serotonin reuptake inhibitors, may provide benefit. Reassurance should also be provided, as many arousal parasomnias decline in frequency as the child enters adolescence.

Adolescent (12–18 Years of Age)

Prevalence and characteristics of sleep disorders

As an individual enters adolescence, there is generally a phase delay in the circadian timing system. This delay may be caused by teenagers' desire for autonomy, their peer culture and social expectations, academic demands, employment opportunities, as well as extracurricular activities. This disruption of the circadian timing system can result in circadian rhythm disorders. Delayed sleep phase syndrome (DSPS) is the most commonly seen circadian rhythm disorder in adolescence. The diagnostic criteria for DSPS is highlighted in **Box 4**. If the patients' bedtime is

Box 4
Diagnostic criteria for circadian rhythm sleep disorder, delayed-sleep-phase type

1. There is a delay in the phase of the major sleep period in relation to the desired sleep time and wake-up time, as evidenced by a chronic or recurrent complaint of inability to fall asleep at a desired conventional clock time together with the inability to awaken at a desired and socially acceptable time.
2. When allowed to choose their preferred schedule, patients will exhibit normal sleep quality and duration for age and maintain a delayed, but stable, phase of entrainment to the 24-hour sleep-wake pattern.
3. Sleep log or actigraphy monitoring (including sleep diary) for at least 7 days demonstrates a stable delay in the timing of the habitual sleep period. (Note: In addition, a delay in the timing of other circadian rhythms, such as the nadir of the core body temperature rhythm or Dim Light Melatonin Onset, is useful for confirmation of the delayed phase.)
4. The sleep disturbance is not better explained by another current sleep disorder, medical or neurologic disorder, mental disorder, medication use, or substance use disorder.

From American Academy of Sleep Medicine. International classification of sleep disorders. In: Sateia M, editor. Diagnostic and coding manual. 3rd edition. Darien (IL): American Academy of Sleep Medicine; 2014. p. 191; with permission.

consistently delayed while school schedules require an early wake time, the persistent short sleep duration can lead to worsening daytime sleepiness during the day.[17]

It is also important to pay special attention to complaints of daytime sleepiness, as symptoms of narcolepsy typically present in the second decade of life. The pentad of symptoms often seen in narcolepsy includes excessive daytime sleepiness, hypnogogic or hypnopompic hallucinations, cataplexy, sleep paralysis, and sleep fragmentation. The complaint of cataplexy can be subtle, and any complaint of loss of muscle tone of the legs or jaw with emotion should warrant further workup including but not limited to overnight polysomnography followed by multiple sleep latency test. In preparation for these studies, patients should be withdrawn from any drugs that may impact sleep architecture, such as central nervous system stimulants, hypnotics, and antidepressants, for 2 weeks before the study.

Management

The complaint of excessive daytime sleepiness should first be managed by ensuring that patients are obtaining an adequate opportunity for sleep. Studies have shown that timed bright-light therapy can be used to phase shift the human circadian clock. Thus, these patients should be counseled about technology use in the evenings, which may further delay their sleep. Conversely, the use of timed bright light therapy in the morning may serve to phase advance the patients' circadian clock back to an appropriate bedtime. The clinician should take care when prescribing bright-light therapy, as administering bright light at the wrong time may exacerbate rather than alleviate symptoms.

When considering the diagnosis of narcolepsy, it is essential to ensure that an accurate diagnosis is made, as patients will require a lifetime of treatment. As the treatment often includes central nervous system stimulants, it is important to also be wary of malingering. The goal in managing narcolepsy is adequate control of the symptoms, and drug treatments are outlined in **Table 4**. There are not any double-blind placebo-controlled trials of medication specifically for the treatment of narcolepsy in children; thus, caution is advised when using these drugs in this patient population.

Table 4
Drugs used in the treatment of narcolepsy

Medication	Dosage
Treatment of excessive daytime sleepiness and cataplexy	
Sodium oxybate	2.25–9.0 g/night
Treatment of excessive daytime sleepiness	
Caffeine	100 mg
Modafinil	100–600 mg
Armodafinil	150–600 mg
Methylphenidate	15–100 mg
Amphetamine	15–60 mg
Dextroamphetamine	15–60 mg
Methamphetamine	15–100 mg
Treatment of cataplexy	
Venlafaxine	75–150 mg
Citalopram	10–40 mg
Paroxetine	10–40 mg
Fluoxetine	20–80 mg
Protriptyline	75–125 mg
Clomipramine	75–125 mg
Imipramine	75–125 mg

Planned napping may also provide a therapeutic benefit in some patients.

Middle-Aged Adults (18–60 Years of Age)

Prevalence and characteristics of sleep disorders

In adults, 3 commonly encountered sleep disorders are insomnia, sleep apnea, and RLS. The diagnostic characteristics of these disorders are described in **Box 5**. Of these 3 sleep disorders, insomnia is by far the most prevalent complaint and is thought to occur in up to 30% of the population. Of the various forms of insomnia, psychophysiological insomnia has the highest in-clinic prevalence rate of 12% to 15%.[18] As reported by Spielman,[19] chronic insomnia is posited to occur because of predisposing, precipitating, and perpetuating factors. Biopsychosocial factors may predispose an individual to the development of insomnia, which may be brought about by an inciting event; the insomnia may become chronic

Box 5
Diagnostic criteria for insomnia, sleep apnea, and RLS

Insomnia

Criteria 1 to 6 must be met

1. The patient reports, or the patient's parent or caregiver observes, one or more of the following:
   a. Difficulty initiating sleep
   b. Difficulty maintaining sleep
   c. Waking up earlier than desired
   d. Resistance to going to bed on appropriate schedule
   e. Difficulty sleeping without parent or caregiver intervention
2. The patient reports, or the patient's parent or caregiver observes, one or more of the following related to the nighttime sleep difficulty:
   a. Fatigue/malaise
   b. Attention, concentration, or memory impairment
   c. Impaired social, family, occupational, or academic performance
   d. Mood disturbance/irritability
   e. Daytime sleepiness
   f. Behavioral problems (eg, hyperactivity, impulsivity, aggression)
   g. Reduced motivation/energy/initiative
   h. Proneness for errors/accidents
   i. Concerns about or dissatisfaction with sleep
3. The reported sleep/wake complaints cannot be explained purely by inadequate opportunity (ie, enough time is allotted for sleep) or inadequate circumstances (ie, the environment is safe, dark, quiet, and comfortable) for sleep
4. The sleep disturbance and associated daytime symptoms occur at least 3 times per week.
5. The sleep disturbance and associated daytime symptoms have been present for at least 3 months.
6. The sleep/wake difficulty is not better explained by another sleep disorder.

OSA

(1 and 2) or 3 satisfy the criteria

1. The presence of one or more of the following:
   a. The patient complains of sleepiness, nonrestorative sleep, fatigue, or insomnia symptoms.
   b. The patient wakes with breath holding, gasping, or choking.
   c. The bed partner or other observer reports habitual snoring, breathing interruptions, or both during the patient's sleep.
   d. The patient has been diagnosed with hypertension, a mood disorder, cognitive dysfunction, coronary artery disease, stroke, congestive heart failure, atrial fibrillation, or type 2 diabetes mellitus.

2. Polysomnography (PSG) or Out of Center Sleep Testing demonstrates
   a. Five or more predominantly obstructive respiratory events (obstructive and mixed apneas, hypopneas, or respiratory effort–related arousals [RERAs]) per hour of sleep during a PSG or per hour of monitoring (Out of Center Sleep Testing)

OR

3. PSG or OCST1 demonstrates
   a. Fifteen or more predominantly obstructive respiratory events (apneas, hypopneas, or RERAs) per hour of sleep during a PSG or per hour of monitoring (Out of Center Sleep Testing)

RLS

Criteria 1 to 3 must be met

1. There is an urge to move the legs, usually accompanied by or thought to be caused by uncomfortable and unpleasant sensations in the legs; these symptoms must
   a. Begin or worsen during periods of rest or inactivity, such as lying down or sitting
   b. Be partially or totally relieved by movement, such as walking or stretching, at least as long as the activity continues and
   c. Occur exclusively or predominantly in the evening or night rather than during the day
2. The aforementioned features are not solely accounted for as symptoms of another medical or a behavioral condition (eg, leg cramps, positional discomfort, myalgia, venous stasis, leg edema, arthritis, habitual foot tapping).
3. The symptoms of RLS cause concern, distress, sleep disturbance, or impairment in mental, physical, social, occupational, educational, behavioral, or other important areas of functioning.

From American Academy of Sleep Medicine. International classification of sleep disorders. In: Sateia M, editor. Diagnostic and coding manual. 3rd edition. Darien (IL): American Academy of Sleep Medicine; 2014; with permission.

if a particular perpetuating factor is allowed to persist.

OSA is also a common disease encountered in this population. The Wisconsin Sleep Cohort Study estimated that the population prevalence of OSA was 9% in women and 24% in men using the current definition of an apnea-hypopnea index greater than 5.[20] Although the prevalence of OSA is generally more common in men than in women, the prevalence of OSA in women seems to increase significantly after menopause. The risk factors for OSA include obesity, family history, and craniofacial structure caused by ethnicity.

Finally, RLS may also be encountered in this patient population. The RLS Epidemiology, Symptoms, and Treatment general population study interviewed a total of 16,202 adults and found a prevalence of 2.7% for clinically significant RLS (frequency at least twice a week with moderate distress).[21] When evaluating patients for RLS, there are several pearls to keep in mind. The use of polysomnography is not indicated, as the diagnosis can be made by history alone. It is also important to differentiate RLS from periodic limb movements of sleep (PLMS). Although PLMS can be present in up to 80% of patients with RLS, the presence of PLMS does not necessarily indicate a diagnosis of RLS unless the diagnostic criterion is met.

Management

Insomnia can generally be managed using pharmacologic treatment, behavioral therapy, or both. About 10% of patients with chronic insomnia use prescription medication to promote sleep. Benzodiazepines and nonbenzodiazepine receptor agonists are approved medications that can be used for the treatment of insomnia. Cognitive behavioral therapy for insomnia (CBT-I) is a multicomponent model of therapy that has been effective in the treatment of insomnia. The primary components include stimulus control and sleep restriction but may also include sleep hygiene education, relaxation techniques, and cognitive restructuring. Morin and colleagues[22] demonstrated that combining CBT-I with pharmacologic therapy was also effective in treating insomnia.

There are several treatment options for the treatment of OSA. Continuous positive airway pressure (CPAP) is considered the gold standard therapy. However, CPAP compliance estimates range between 17% and 71%.[23] Given the poor adherence to CPAP use, alternative treatment options have emerged. The use of an oral appliance, which protrudes a patient's mandible forward, has been shown to reduce snoring and can be an effective treatment of OSA.[24] Several upper airway surgeries, including maxillomandibular advancement and uvulopalatopharyngoplasty, may also reduce the disease severity by as much as 87% and 33%, respectively.[25,26] Weight loss should also be encouraged, as a 10% reduction in weight can result in a 26% reduction in the severity of OSA.[27]

A consensus-based algorithm has been developed for the treatment of RLS and is summarized in **Fig. 1**.[28] For intermittent RLS, mentally stimulating activities (word puzzles, writing, reading), exercise, and massage may help patients to cope with symptoms. Symptoms that occur daily may warrant pharmacologic intervention. The mainstay of RLS therapy has traditionally been dopaminergic agents, such as pramipexole or ropinirole. More recently, the rotigotine transdermal patch has also been available as a treatment option. The limiting factor for long-term use of these agents is augmentation of RLS symptoms. Dopaminergic agents may also increase the risk for impulse control disorders. Anticonvulsants, hypnotics, and opiates may also be considered in cases of refractory RLS.

Elderly (>60 Years of Age)

Prevalence and characteristics of sleep disorders

There is a high prevalence of reported sleep disturbances in older adults. More than 50% of noninstitutionalized adults older than 65 years report chronic disruption of sleep.[29] Foley and colleagues[29] reported epidemiologic findings of up to 43% of older adults with complaints of initiating or maintaining sleep. There are many factors that can contribute to sleep disturbances in the older adult (**Table 5**). Often, sleep complaints may be caused by behavioral/environmental issues. Many individuals older than 65 years are retired, which can reduce the need for a consistent sleep-and-wake schedule. However, medical disorders, psychiatric disorders, sleep disorders and medications can also contribute to sleep complaints. Additionally, patients who are institutionalized may have a greater risk of sleep disturbance because of the infrequent ambulation, social isolation, and

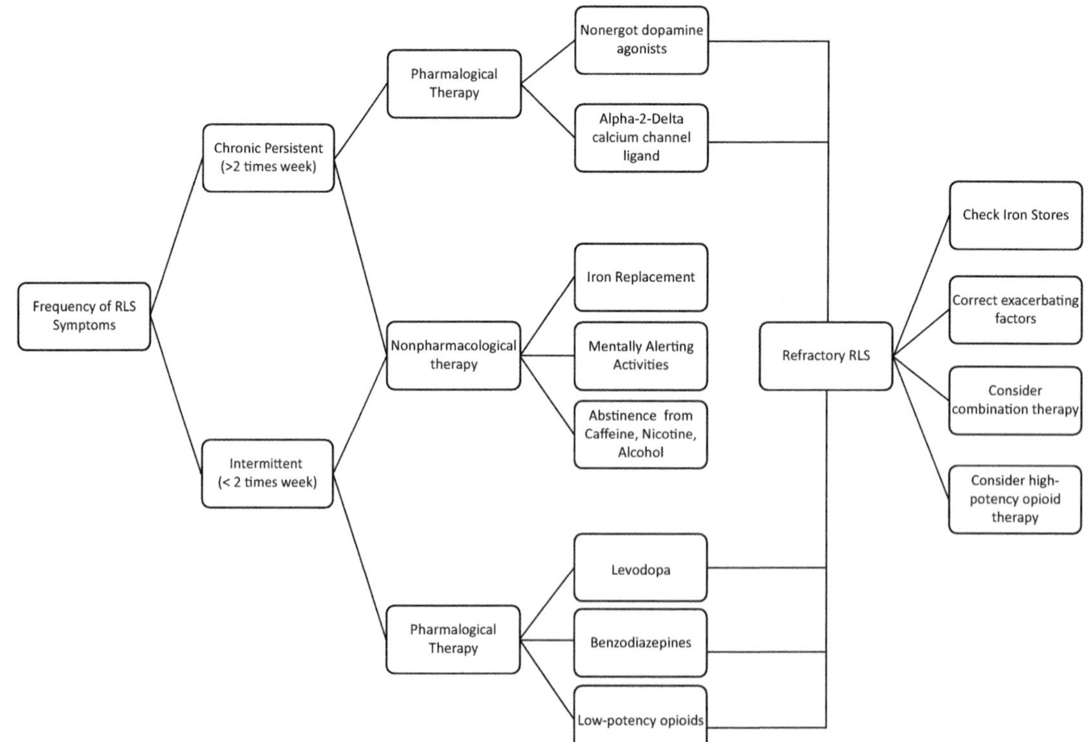

Fig. 1. Management of RLS. (*Adapted from* Silber MH, Becker PM, Earley C, et al, for the Medical Advisory Board of the Willis-Ekbom Disease Foundation. Willis-Ekbom disease foundation revised consensus statement on the management of restless legs syndrome. Mayo Clinic Proc 2013;88(9):977–86.)

Table 5
Causes of sleep disruption in older adults

Cause	Example
Behavioral	Retirement reducing need for consistent sleep/wake schedule Napping
Medical	Chronic pain Chronic cardiac or pulmonary disease
Psychiatric	Depression
Medication	Diuretics leading to nocturnal awakening
Sleep disorders	OSA REM behavior disorder RLS

decreased daily activity. Persistent sleep disruption and deprivation may contribute to a higher incidence of falls in this patient population.

Medicare claims data can provide some perspective on common health complaints among individuals aged 65 years and older (**Fig. 2**). Many of these disease processes have a bidirectional relationship with sleep disruption, as many can lead to sleep disruption and conversely sleep disruption can influence the disease status. In addition, patients with these medical disorders have a higher prevalence of sleep disorders. Twenty-five percent of patients with rheumatoid arthritis have symptoms consistent with RLS.[30] Patients with chronic kidney disease on hemodialysis have been found to have a higher prevalence of OSA, RLS, insomnia, and daytime sleepiness.[31–33]

Medications also have a profound effect on sleep. Polypharmacy including prescription and over-the-counter medications is common in older adults. Population-based studies have shown that 46% of adults older than 65 years take at least 5 medications a day.[34] It is important to review the patients' medication history, as medications may be sedating, activating, or exacerbate their existing medical or sleep disorder (**Box 6**). Antihistamine, antidepressants, caffeine, alcohol, and nicotine can all exacerbate RLS symptoms. Agents such as hypnotics, opiates, and muscle relaxants may worsen sleep-disordered breathing.

Management

Given the bidirectional relationship between many medical disorders and sleep, it is vital to ensure that these disorders are managed optimally. Indeed, treating the underlying disorder may improve sleep complaints, and treating sleep complaints may improve symptoms of the medical disorder. For example, CBT-I has been shown to improve sleep and decrease pain in individuals with osteoarthritis and comorbid insomnia.[35] In individuals with gastroesophageal reflux disease, acid-suppression therapy can lead to a reduction in nocturnal heartburn symptoms and sleep disruption and has been shown to improve next-day work performance.[36]

The medication list should be reviewed periodically. The effects of as-needed medications on sleep and wake should be considered and used judiciously. The practitioner may consider dosing medications that may be activating away from the sleep period and conversely be aware of medications that may promote sleepiness during the day. Behavioral treatments can also be useful in this patient population. Increasing bright-light exposure and scheduling structured activities

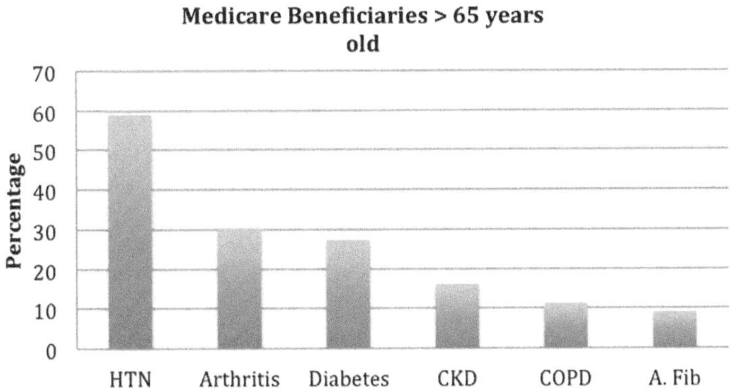

Fig. 2. Common health complaints of individuals aged 65 years and older. A. Fib, atrial fibrillation; CKD, chronic kidney disease; COPD, chronic obstructive pulmonary disease; HTN, hypertension. (*Data from* Centers for Medicare and Medicaid Services. Geographic variation public use file. Available at: http://www.cms.gov/Research-Statistics-Data-and-Systems/Statistics-Trends-and-Reports/Medicare-Geographic-Variation/GV_PUF.html. Accessed January 8, 2014.)

Box 6
Medications that disrupt sleep

Sedating medications
Anticholinergic agents
Antihistamines
Antispasmodics
Antipsychotics
Antiemetics
Antiparkinsonian drugs
Sedating antidepressants
Opiates

Activating medications
OTC agents containing pseudoephedrine
Caffeine
Beta agonists
Corticosteroids
Theophylline
Activating antidepressants
Methylphenidate
Modafinil

Abbreviation: OTC, over the counter.

during the day may help in the regulation of circadian rhythms.

SUMMARY

Sleep is a dynamic process that is changing throughout the lifespan. Understanding normal physiologic changes and factors that can disrupt sleep can aid in the evaluation and management of sleep complaints. There are also several questionnaires, surveys, and diagnostic tools to supplement the clinical evaluation. Understanding sleep disorders that are prevalent in different stages of life can help with narrowing the possible differential diagnoses. Sleep disorders are not an inevitable part of aging, and appropriate treatment can result in significant improvement in quality of life for patients of all ages.

REFERENCES

1. Ohayon MM, Carskadon MA, Guilleminault C, et al. Meta-analysis of quantitative sleep parameters from childhood to old age in healthy individuals: developing normative sleep values across the human lifespan. Sleep 2004;27(7):1255–73.
2. Buysse DJ, Browman KE, Monk TH, et al. Napping and 24-hour sleep/wake patterns in healthy elderly and young adults. J Am Geriatr Soc 1992;40(8):779–86.
3. National Sleep Foundation. 2003 Sleep in America Poll. National Sleep Foundation Website.
4. Metz ME, Bunnell DE. Napping and sleep disturbances in the elderly. Fam Pract Res J 1990;10(1):47–56.
5. Johns MW. A new method for measuring daytime sleepiness: the Epworth sleepiness scale. Sleep 1991;14(6):540–5.
6. Buysse DJ, Reynolds CF 3rd, Monk TH, et al. The Pittsburgh Sleep Quality Index: a new instrument for psychiatric practice and research. Psychiatry Res 1989;28(2):193–213.
7. Owens JA, Dalzell V. Use of the 'BEARS' sleep screening tool in a pediatric residents' continuity clinic: a pilot study. Sleep Med 2005;6(1):63–9.
8. Owens JA, Spirito A, McGuinn M. The Children's Sleep Habits Questionnaire (CSHQ): psychometric properties of a survey instrument for school-aged children. Sleep 2000;23(8):1043–51.
9. Morgenthaler T, Alessi C, Friedman L, et al. Practice parameters for the use of actigraphy in the assessment of sleep and sleep disorders: an update for 2007. Sleep 2007;30(4):519–29.
10. Littner MR, Kushida C, Wise M, et al. Practice parameters for clinical use of the multiple sleep latency test and the maintenance of wakefulness test. Sleep 2005;28(1):113–21.
11. Blader JC, Koplewicz HS, Abikoff H, et al. Sleep problems of elementary school children. A community survey. Arch Pediatr Adolesc Med 1997;151(5):473–80.
12. Kahn A, Van de Merckt C, Rebuffat E, et al. Sleep problems in healthy preadolescents. Pediatrics 1989;84(3):542–6.
13. Rona RJ, Li L, Gulliford MC, et al. Disturbed sleep: effects of sociocultural factors and illness. Arch Dis Child 1998;78(1):20–5.
14. Owens JA, Spirito A, McGuinn M, et al. Sleep habits and sleep disturbance in elementary school-aged children. J Dev Behav Pediatr 2000;21(1):27–36.
15. Moore M, Allison D, Rosen CL. A review of pediatric nonrespiratory sleep disorders. Chest 2006;130:1252–62.
16. Morgenthaler TI, Owens J, Alessi C, et al. Practice parameters for behavioral treatment of bedtime problems and night wakings in infants and young children. Sleep 2006;29(10):1277–81.
17. Carskadon MA. Patterns of sleep and sleepiness in adolescents. Pediatrician 1990;17(1):5–12.
18. American Academy of Sleep Medicine. International classification of sleep disorders. 2nd edition. Diagnostic and coding manual. Westchester, Illinois: American Academy of Sleep Medicine; 2005.
19. Spielman AJ, Glovinsky PB. The varied nature of insomnia. In: Hauri P, editor. Case studies in insomnia. New York: Plenum Press; 1991. p. 1–3.

20. Young T, Palta M, Dempsey J, et al. The occurrence of sleep-disordered breathing among middle-aged adults. N Engl J Med 1993;328(17):1230–5.
21. Allen RP, Walters AS, Montplaisir J, et al. Restless legs syndrome prevalence and impact: REST general population study. Arch Intern Med 2005;165(11):1286–92.
22. Morin CM, Vallieres A, Guay B, et al. Cognitive behavioral therapy, singly and combined with medication, for persistent insomnia: a randomized controlled trial. JAMA 2009;301(19):2005–15.
23. Weaver TE, Grunstein RR. Adherence to continuous positive airway pressure therapy: the challenge to effective treatment. Proc Am Thorac Soc 2008;5(2):173–8.
24. Li W, Xiao L, Hu J. The comparison of CPAP and oral appliances in treatment of patients with OSA: a systematic review and meta-analysis. Respir Care 2013;58(7):1184–95.
25. Caples SM, Rowley JA, Prinsell JR, et al. Surgical modifications of the upper airway for obstructive sleep apnea in adults: a systematic review and meta-analysis. Sleep 2010;33(10):1396–407.
26. Holty JE, Guilleminault C. Maxillomandibular advancement for the treatment of obstructive sleep apnea: a systematic review and meta-analysis. Sleep Med Rev 2010;14(5):287–97.
27. Peppard PE, Young T, Palta M, et al. Longitudinal study of moderate weight change and sleep-disordered breathing. JAMA 2000;284(23):3015–21.
28. Silber MH, Becker PM, Earley C, et al, Medical Advisory Board of the Willis-Ekbom Disease Foundation. Willis-Ekbom Disease Foundation revised consensus statement on the management of restless legs syndrome. Mayo Clin Proc 2013;88(9):977–86.
29. Foley DJ, Monjan AA, Brown SL, et al. Sleep complaints among elderly persons: an epidemiologic study of three communities. Sleep 1995;18(6):425–32.
30. Salih AM, Gray RE, Mills KR, et al. A clinical, serological and neurophysiological study of restless legs syndrome in rheumatoid arthritis. Br J Rheumatol 1994;33(1):60–3.
31. Hanly PJ, Pierratos A. Improvement of sleep apnea in patients with chronic renal failure who undergo nocturnal hemodialysis. N Engl J Med 2001;344(2):102–7.
32. Parker KP. Sleep disturbances in dialysis patients. Sleep Med Rev 2003;7(2):131–43.
33. Williams SW, Tell GS, Zheng B, et al. Correlates of sleep behavior among hemodialysis patients. The kidney outcomes prediction and evaluation (KOPE) study. Am J Nephrol 2002;22(1):18–28.
34. Kaufman DW, Kelly JP, Rosenberg L, et al. Recent patterns of medication use in the ambulatory adult population of the United States: the Slone survey. JAMA 2002;287(3):337–44.
35. Vitiello MV, Rybarczyk B, Von Korff M, et al. Cognitive behavioral therapy for insomnia improves sleep and decreases pain in older adults with co-morbid insomnia and osteoarthritis. J Clin Sleep Med 2009;5(4):355–62.
36. Johnson DA, Orr WC, Crawley JA, et al. Effect of esomeprazole on nighttime heartburn and sleep quality in patients with GERD: a randomized, placebo-controlled trial. Am J Gastroenterol 2005;100(9):1914–22.

Index

Note: Page numbers of article titles are in **boldface** type.

Sleep Med Clin 9 (2014) 585–589
http://dx.doi.org/10.1016/S1556-407X(14)00113-1
1556-407X/14/$ – see front matter

United States Postal Service

Statement of Ownership, Management, and Circulation (All Periodicals Publications Except Requestor Publications)

1. Publication Title	2. Publication Number	3. Filing Date
Sleep Medicine Clinics	0 2 5 - 0 5 3	9/14/14
4. Issue Frequency: Mar, Jun, Sep, Dec	5. Number of Issues Published Annually: 4	6. Annual Subscription Price: $195.00

7. Complete Mailing Address of Known Office of Publication (*Not printer*) (*Street, city, county, state, and ZIP+4®*)

Elsevier Inc.
360 Park Avenue South
New York, NY 10010-1710

Contact Person: Stephen R. Bushing
Telephone (Include area code): 215-239-3688

8. Complete Mailing Address of Headquarters or General Business Office of Publisher (*Not printer*)

Elsevier Inc., 360 Park Avenue South, New York, NY 10010-1710

9. Full Names and Complete Mailing Addresses of Publisher, Editor, and Managing Editor (*Do not leave blank*)

Publisher (*Name and complete mailing address*)

Linda Belfus, Elsevier, Inc., 1600 John F. Kennedy Blvd. Suite 1800, Philadelphia, PA 19103-2899

Editor (*Name and complete mailing address*)

Patrick Manley, Elsevier, Inc., 1600 John F. Kennedy Blvd. Suite 1800, Philadelphia, PA 19103-2899

Managing Editor (*Name and complete mailing address*)

Adrianne Brigido, Elsevier, Inc., 1600 John F. Kennedy Blvd. Suite 1800, Philadelphia, PA 19103-2899

10. Owner (*Do not leave blank. If the publication is owned by a corporation, give the name and address of the corporation immediately followed by the names and addresses of all stockholders owning or holding 1 percent or more of the total amount of stock. If not owned by a corporation, give the names and addresses of the individual owners. If owned by a partnership or other unincorporated firm, give its name and address as well as those of each individual owner. If the publication is published by a nonprofit organization, give its name and address.*)

Full Name	Complete Mailing Address
Wholly owned subsidiary of	1600 John F. Kennedy Blvd, Ste. 1800
Reed/Elsevier, US holdings	Philadelphia, PA 19103-2899

11. Known Bondholders, Mortgagees, and Other Security Holders Owning or Holding 1 Percent or More of Total Amount of Bonds, Mortgages, or Other Securities. If none, check box → None

Full Name	Complete Mailing Address
N/A	

12. Tax Status (*For completion by nonprofit organizations authorized to mail at nonprofit rates*) (*Check one*)
The purpose, function, and nonprofit status of this organization and the exempt status for federal income tax purposes:
Has Not Changed During Preceding 12 Months
Has Changed During Preceding 12 Months (*Publisher must submit explanation of change with this statement*)

PS Form 3526, August 2012 (Page 1 of 3 (Instructions Page 3)) PSN 7530-01-000-9931 **PRIVACY NOTICE:** See our Privacy policy in www.usps.com

13. Publication Title: Sleep Medicine Clinics
14. Issue Date for Circulation Data Below: June 2014

15. Extent and Nature of Circulation		Average No. Copies Each Issue During Preceding 12 Months	No. Copies of Single Issue Published Nearest to Filing Date
a. Total Number of Copies (*Net press run*)		524	488
b. Paid Circulation (By Mail and Outside the Mail)	(1) Mailed Outside-County Paid Subscriptions Stated on PS Form 3541. (*Include paid distribution above nominal rate, advertiser's proof copies, and exchange copies*)	359	322
	(2) Mailed In-County Paid Subscriptions Stated on PS Form 3541 (*Include paid distribution above nominal rate, advertiser's proof copies, and exchange copies*)		
	(3) Paid Distribution Outside the Mails Including Sales Through Dealers and Carriers, Street Vendors, Counter Sales, and Other Paid Distribution Outside USPS®	28	28
	(4) Paid Distribution by Other Classes Mailed Through the USPS (e.g. First-Class Mail®)		
c. Total Paid Distribution (*Sum of 15b (1), (2), (3), and (4)*) ►		387	350
d. Free or Nominal Rate Distribution (By Mail and Outside the Mail)	(1) Free or Nominal Rate Outside-County Copies Included on PS Form 3541	59	63
	(2) Free or Nominal Rate In-County Copies Included on PS Form 3541		
	(3) Free or Nominal Rate Copies Mailed at Other Classes Through the USPS (e.g. First-Class Mail)		
	(4) Free or Nominal Rate Distribution Outside the Mail (Carriers or other means)		
e. Total Free or Nominal Rate Distribution (Sum of 15d (1), (2), (3) and (4)		59	63
f. Total Distribution (Sum of 15c and 15e) ►		446	413
g. Copies not Distributed (See instructions to publishers #4 (page #3)) ►		78	75
h. Total (Sum of 15f and g)		524	488
i. Percent Paid (15c divided by 15f times 100) ►		86.77%	84.75%
16. Total circulation includes electronic copies. Report circulation on PS Form 3526-X worksheet. ►			

17. Publication of Statement of Ownership
If the publication is a general publication, publication of this statement is required. Will be printed in the December 2014 issue of this publication.

18. Signature and Title of Editor, Publisher, Business Manager, or Owner
Stephen R. Bushing – Inventory Distribution Coordinator
Date: September 14, 2014

I certify that all information furnished on this form is true and complete. I understand that anyone who furnishes false or misleading information on this form or who omits material or information requested on the form may be subject to criminal sanctions (including fines and imprisonment) and/or civil sanctions (including civil penalties).

PS Form 3526, August 2012 (Page 2 of 3)

Printed and bound by CPI Group (UK) Ltd, Croydon, CR0 4YY
03/10/2024
01040376-0012

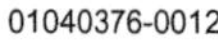